Workshops in

Fluid and Electrolyte Disorders

Workshops in
Fluid and Electrolyte Disorders

Edited by

Harold M. Szerlip, M.D.

Associate Professor and Associate Chairman
Department of Medicine
Tulane University School of Medicine
Chief
Tulane Medical Service
Charity Hospital
New Orleans, Louisiana

Stanley Goldfarb, M.D.

Clinical Professor
Department of Medicine
University of Pennsylvania School of Medicine
Vice President for Patient Care, Education, and Research
Graduate Health System
Philadelphia, Pennsylvania

Churchill Livingstone
New York, Edinburgh, London, Madrid, Melbourne, Tokyo

Library of Congress Cataloging-in-Publication Data

Workshops in fluid and electrolyte disorders : a practical and case
    -oriented approach / edited by Harold M. Szerlip, Stanley Goldfarb.
        p.   cm.
    Includes bibliographical references and index.
    ISBN 0-443-08791-1
    1. Body fluid disorders   2. Water-electrolyte disorders.
    I. Szerlip, Harold M.   II. Goldfarb, Stanley.
    [DNLM: 1. Water-Electrolyte Imbalance—outlines.   2. Water
    -Electrolyte Imbalance—examination questions.   WD 200 W926 1993]
    RC630.W67 1993
    616.3'9—dc20
    DNLM/DLC
    for Library of Congress   93-11387
                                                                                CIP

© **Churchill Livingstone Inc. 1993**

Distributed in the United Kingdom by Churchill Livingstone, Robert Stevenson House, 1–3 Baxter's Place, Leith Walk, Edinburgh EH1 3AF, and by associated companies, branches, and representatives throughout the world.

Accurate indications, adverse reactions, and dosage schedules for drugs are provided in this book, but it is possible that they may change. The reader is urged to review the package information data of the manufacturers of the medications mentioned.

The Publishers have made every effort to trace the copyright holders for borrowed material. If they have inadvertently overlooked any, they will be pleased to make the necessary arrangements at the first opportunity.

Copy Editor: *Elizabeth Bowman-Schulman*
Production Supervisor: *Patricia McFadden*
Cover Design: *Paul Moran*

Printed in the United States of America

First published in 1993   7 6 5 4 3 2 1

To Marjorie, Aaron, and David who have always supported me;
and to all the students who have taught me
as much as I taught them.   H.M.S.

To Rayna, Rachael, and Michael whom I love and to
Donna Kern McCurdy who inspired this approach
to fluid and electrolyte disorders.   S.G.

Contributors

Anthony Bleyer, M.D.
Instructor, Division of Nephrology, Department of Internal Medicine, Bowman Gray School of Medicine of Wake Forest University, Winston-Salem, North Carolina

Michael Choi, M.D.
Post-Doctoral Fellow, Renal-Electrolyte Division, Department of Medicine, University of Pennsylvania School of Medicine, Philadelphia, Pennsylvania

Malcolm Cox, M.D.
Professor and Vice-Chairman, Department of Medicine, University of Pennsylvania School of Medicine; Chief, Medical Service, Philadelphia Veterans Affairs Medical Center, Philadelphia, Pennsylvania

Theodore M. Danoff, M.D., Ph.D.
Post-Doctoral Fellow, Renal-Electrolyte Division, Department of Medicine, University of Pennsylvania School of Medicine, Philadelphia, Pennsylvania

George M. Feldman, M.D.
Associate Professor, Department of Medicine and Physiology, Virginia Commonwealth University Medical College of Virginia School of Medicine; Chief, Renal Section, McGuire Veterans Affairs Medical Center; Attending Physician and Consultant, Division of Nephrology, Department of Internal Medicine, Medical College of Virginia Hospitals, Richmond, Virginia

Pedro C. Fernandez, M.D.
Professor, Department of Medicine, Medical College of Pennsylvania; Adjunct Associate Professor, Renal-Electrolyte Division, Department of Medicine, University of Pennsylvania School of Medicine, Philadelphia, Pennsylvania

Robert A. Gayner, M.D.
Post-Doctoral Fellow, Renal-Electrolyte Division, Department of Medicine, University of Pennsylvania School of Medicine, Philadelphia, Pennsylvania

Stanley Goldfarb, M.D.
Clinical Professor, Department of Medicine, University of Pennsylvania School of Medicine; Vice President for Patient Care, Education, and Research, Graduate Health System, Philadelphia, Pennsylvania

Gail Morrison, M.D.
Associate Professor, Renal-Electrolyte Division, Department of Medicine, and Associate Chairman, Department of Medicine, University of Pennsylvania School of Medicine; Associate Dean, University of Pennsylvania School of Medicine, Philadelphia, Pennsylvania

Eric G. Neilson, M.D.
Professor, Department of Medicine, University of Pennsylvania School of Medicine; Chief, Renal-Electrolyte Division, Hospital of the University of Pennsylvania, Philadelphia, Pennsylvania

Kumar Sharma, M.D.
Post-Doctoral Fellow, Renal-Electrolyte Division, Department of Medicine, University of Pennsylvania School of Medicine, Philadelphia, Pennsylvania

Fuad Shihab, M.D.
Assistant Professor, Division of Nephrology, Department of Medicine, University of Utah School of Medicine, Salt Lake City, Utah

Harold M. Szerlip, M.D.
Associate Professor and Associate Chairman, Department of Medicine, Tulane University School of Medicine; Chief, Tulane Medical Service, Charity Hospital, New Orleans, Louisiana

Fuad N. Ziyadeh, M.D.
Assistant Professor, Renal-Electrolyte Division, Department of Medicine, University of Pennsylvania School of Medicine, Philadelphia, Pennsylvania

Preface

Superficially, it might be said that the function of the kidneys is to make urine; but in a more considered view one can say that the kidneys make the stuff of philosophy itself.

Homer W. Smith
From Fish to Philosopher (1953)

The explosion of medical information has made it difficult, if not impossible, for students of medicine to keep abreast of the ever increasing amount of knowledge. What has become clear in medical education, however, is that memorization of facts is less important than the ability to solve problems. Problem solving requires an understanding of basic concepts that serve not only as the foundation for future learning but also as the keystone in the approach to the patient. In no area of medicine is the ability to approach patient problems as well grounded in basic principles of physiology as the study of fluid and electrolyte disorders. It is this physiologic infrastructure that makes the teaching of nephrology ideally suited for problem-based learning.

There are many excellent textbooks of nephrology aimed at students and housestaff. *Workshops in Fluid and Electrolyte Disorders* is not meant to replace or compete with any of the standard texts, but rather to serve as a companion. It is designed to be used by students as an added learning experience during their pathophysiology course or clinical clerkship in medicine or nephrology. We believe it will also be beneficial to housestaff for board examination review.

This text is based on a long-running and well-received pathophysiology course at the University of Pennsylvania School of Medicine that predates the current popularity of problem-based learning. This course has been exported to numerous medical schools by former University of Pennsylvania renal faculty and fellows, and its offspring has helped train many of today's nephrologists. It was the many rave reviews the course received from students that served as the impetus to take this material from the classroom to the publisher. In this course the students are taught the basic concepts of renal pathophysiology and are then asked to apply these concepts to a series of patient problems.

The text follows a similar approach. Each chapter begins with a brief outline of the important principles. General readings are given if more in-depth knowledge is desired. This introduction is followed by a case study (or studies) and a set of patient problems with questions designed to guide the student through the important aspects of each case. Comprehensive answers are then provided. Cases have been designed to stand alone. Thus the reader may review a single case, a single chapter, multiple chapters, or the entire book. While this leads to some duplication of material, we believe that this too is educationally valuable.

We hope readers of this text find it a novel and enjoyable way to gain an understanding of fluid and electrolyte disorders. Writing it certainly was an enjoyable experience for all the contributors.

Harold M. Szerlip, M.D.
Stanley Goldfarb, M.D.

Contents

1

Sodium and Volume Homeostasis

Michael Choi
Harold M. Szerlip

BODY FLUID COMPARTMENTS

Total Body Water

Water is the major constituent of the body and accounts for approximately 60% of body weight. Two-thirds of total body water (TBW) is concentrated in the intracellular fluid (ICF) compartment and the remaining third in the extracellular fluid (ECF) compartment. Most cell membranes are freely permeable to water, and thus at steady state the osmolality of these two compartments is equal. A change in osmolality of one compartment results in the passive movement of water from the area of lower osmolality to the area of higher osmolality. In the ECF, the principal solute is sodium; in the ICF, the major solute is potassium.

Extracellular Fluid Compartment

The ECF compartment is partitioned by vascular endothelium into an intravascular compartment, which contains circulating plasma, and an interstitial compartment that bathes all cells. A dynamic equilibrium exists between these two compartments. There is a constant flow of fluid across the capillary bed from the intravascular to the interstitial space, and an equal flow of fluid from the interstitial space back into the intravascular space through the lymphatic system. The movement of fluid across the capillary membrane is determined by the permeability of the membrane and the net difference between the hydrostatic pressure gradient, which drives fluid out of the intravascular space and the oncotic pressure gradient, which holds fluid within the intravascular space.

Total Body Sodium

Sodium is the major osmotically active solute within the ECF compartment and thus dictates the distribution of water between the ICF and the ECF spaces. Because Na is relatively confined to the ECF space by active extrusion from cells by Na^+, K^+-ATPase, total body Na content

1

determines the volume of the ECF space. It is important not to confuse disorders of Na content with disorders of Na concentration. The latter are problems in water balance and not Na homeostasis.

SODIUM HOMEOSTASIS

Sodium Balance

Total body Na content depends on the balance between Na intake and excretion. When excretion is greater than intake, Na balance is negative and the ECF volume shrinks; conversely, when excretion is less than intake, Na balance is positive and the ECF volume expands. Sodium intake varies according to diet and the parenteral administration of medications or fluids that contain sodium. Sodium is excreted primarily by the kidney; negligible losses also occur through the gastrointestinal tract and the skin. In certain pathologic conditions like diarrhea or diffuse burns, however, extrarenal losses of Na can be significant.

Renal Na excretion is the ultimate arbiter of total body sodium—and therefore extracellular and intravascular volume—because the kidney can adjust to a wide range of Na intakes and because nonrenal sodium losses are normally small.

Renal Sodium Excretion Regulation

Although the absolute volume of the intravascular space is an important component of circulatory "fullness," the adequacy of the circulation (more commonly called the effective arterial blood volume or EABV) also is determined by cardiac output and systemic vascular resistance (Fig. 1-1). An intricate array of homeostatic controls monitors and regulates EABV. A fall in EABV results in a compensatory increase in cardiac output, an increase in systemic vascular resistance, and renal Na retention. An increase in EABV has opposite effects. Unfortunately, no readily quantifiable parameter can serve as a direct measurement of EABV, and in certain conditions EABV may be decreased despite ECF volume overload. Therefore, renal Na excretion best reflects the fullness of the circulation. The normal kidney responds to an inadequate EABV by conserving Na, and excretes Na when EABV is increased.

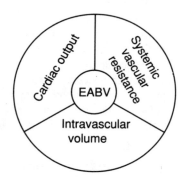

Fig. 1-1. Effective arterial blood volume (EABV) is made up of three components: absolute volume of the intravascular space, cardiac output, and systemic vascular resistance. A change in any one of these parameters without a compensatory change in the others will affect the fullness of the circulation.

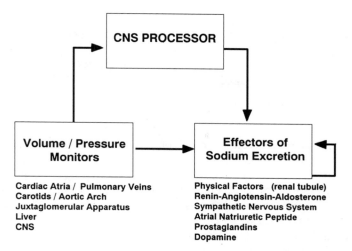

Fig. 1-2. Homeostatic regulation of sodium balance. CNS, central nervous system.

MECHANICS OF SODIUM HOMEOSTASIS

Like any homeostatic system, the system that regulates total body Na content consists of an afferent (sensory) limb, which monitors the functional integrity of the circulation, and an efferent (effector) limb, which controls renal Na excretion (Fig. 1-2).

Volume and Pressure Monitors

Given that the goals of the volume regulatory system are to optimize intravascular volume, arterial pressure, and tissue perfusion, it is not surprising that monitors are located at points ideally suited for sensing volume, pressure, and tissue perfusion.

Low Pressure Sensors

The pulmonary vasculature and cardiac atria contain 75% to 80% of the intravascular volume; this low pressure, high volume system is thus an ideal location for volume sensors. Increased intravascular volume distends the cardiac atria and leads to the release of atrial natriuretic peptide and a decrease in renal sympathetic activity; these both increase renal Na excretion.

High Pressure Sensors

Monitoring of intravascular volume occurs on the venous side of the circulation, but pressure monitoring by necessity must occur on the arterial side of the circulation. The carotid sinuses and aortic arch contain presumptive baroreceptors that monitor arterial pressure. A decline in blood pressure produces an increase in renal sympathetic activity, leading to Na retention.

Juxtaglomerular Apparatus

The JGA located within the kidney is ideally situated to monitor both renal perfusion and solute excretion. The JGA consists of specialized renin-secreting cells in the afferent glomerular arteriole and highly differentiated cells in the distal tubule (the macula densa). Decreased wall tension in the afferent arteriole or decreased salt delivery to the macula densa stimulates the juxtaglomerular cells to release renin. In addition, renin release is also under adrenergic control.

Volume Regulatory Effectors

The kidneys maintain extracellular fluid volume by regulating the reabsorption of Na from the urine through multiple effector systems.

The Proximal Tubule

Luminal Na enters proximal tubular cells through a variety of coupled transporters and is then pumped into the lateral intercellular space by Na^+,K^+-ATPase. Because of the high hydraulic conductivity of the luminal membrane, water quickly follows Na, so that fluid reabsorption occurs isotonically. From the lateral intercellular space, the reabsorbed salt and H_2O can either leak back into the tubule lumen or enter the peritubular capillary network. The magnitude of reabsorption depends on the physical factors (the hydrostatic and oncotic pressure gradients) existing between the peritubular interstitial space and the capillary lumen. An increase in oncotic pressure or a decrease in hydrostatic pressure in the peritubular capillaries augments salt and H_2O uptake by the capillary and decreases backleak into the tubule lumen. Opposite changes in these physical factors result in decreased sodium reabsorption.

Renin-Angiotensin-Aldosterone System

Renin secretion is under multifactorial control. Renin converts angiotensinogen to angiotensin I, which is further metabolized by angiotensin-converting enzyme to angiotensin II (AII). Besides being a vasoconstrictor, AII is a potent antinatriuretic hormone. Angiotensin II directly activates sodium-coupled transport in the proximal tubule, and by preferentially constricting the efferent glomerular arteriole, it also increases the fraction of plasma filtered at the glomerulus. This elevates the oncotic pressure in the postglomerular capillary and thus indirectly increases proximal tubular Na reabsorption. In addition, AII stimulates aldosterone secretion, which enhances reabsorption of Na in the distal tubule.

Sympathetic Nervous System

Sensors responsive to stretch and pressure monitor circulatory fullness and transmit this information to a central nervous system (CNS) processor (e.g., hypothalamus or medulla oblongata), which in turn regulates sympathetic outflow to the kidneys. An extensive adrenergic innervation exists throughout the length of the nephron. Renal denervation blunts renal Na conservation; conversely, stimulation of renal sympathetic nerves increases Na reabsorption by all segments of the nephrons both directly and indirectly (via renin release).

Atrial Natriuretic Peptide

The cardiac atria contain secretory granules that are released into the circulation in response to atrial stretch. Packaged within these granules is a recently characterized peptide, atrial natriuretic peptide (ANP). This peptide increases renal blood flow and glomerular filtration rate, decreases Na reabsorption in the medullary collecting duct, inhibits renin and aldosterone release, and increases the flux of fluid from the intravascular to the interstitial space. These actions all function to decrease the volume of the intravascular space.

Prostaglandins

Prostaglandins are synthesized by a variety of renal cells and have important roles in salt and H_2O excretion. For the most part, prostaglandins act by modulating the effects of other hormones. For example, AII is a potent stimulator of PGE_2 and PGI synthesis; in turn, these eicosanoids counteract the sodium retaining effects of AII. Renal prostaglandin synthesis is increased in states of absolute or effective volume depletion, and serves to maintain glomerular filtration rate and the excretion of salt and water. Inhibition of prostaglandin synthesis under these circumstances can lead to dramatic declines in the glomerular filtration rate and worsening sodium overload.

Dopamine

Both dopamine receptors and dopamine-containing neuronal elements are abundantly present throughout the kidney. Renal dopamine excretion parallels renal Na excretion. Inhibition of dopamine synthesis attenuates the natriuretic response to saline loading, whereas dopamine agonists are natriuretic. Dopamine appears to decrease Na reabsorption in the proximal tubule by inhibiting Na^+,K^+-ATPase activity.

Glomerular Filtration Rate

The amount of sodium presented to the tubule is dependent on the glomerular filtration rate (GFR). Several regulatory mechanisms, however, moderate the role of GFR in renal Na excretion. First, despite fluctuations in renal blood flow, autoregulation prevents major changes in GFR. Second, changes in the filtered load of Na are matched by parallel changes in Na, such that a fixed proportion (rather than an absolute amount) of the filtered load is reabsorbed. This linkage between filtration and reabsorption is called glomerulotubular balance. Thus, an increase in GFR of 10%, which increases the filtered load of Na by several thousand milliequivalents, results in only a 10% increase in Na excretion (i.e., from 100 to 110 mEq). The mechanisms underlying glomerulotubular balance include changes in physical factors and alterations in luminal organic solute delivery. Finally, if the proximal tubule's absorptive capacity is overwhelmed by an increase in the filtered load, the resultant increased solute delivery to the macula densa produces a reflex decrease in filtration rate (tubular glomerular feedback).

CLINICAL ASSESSMENT OF VOLUME STATUS

Disorders of ECF volume homeostasis are divided into two broad categories: Na excess and Na depletion. Although such a classification system is a helpful diagnostic heuristic, it is too simplistic because it does not adequately reflect the physiologic basis for the homeostatic responses that occur. Tissue perfusion is the critical element in any consideration of ECF volume homeostasis, and so it is best to categorize disorders of ECF volume homeostasis based on a tripartite schema that includes assessment of total body Na (ECF volume), intravascular volume, and effective arterial blood volume. These three parameters change in parallel in Na-depleted states. In Na-overload conditions, however, this is not always the case. For example, it is not uncommon to find a decreased EABV (as determined by a low urine Na) despite massive total body Na overload. Fortunately, a careful history and physical examination usually provide sufficient information to classify most disorders of volume homeostasis.

ECF Volume Overload (Increased Total Body Sodium)

The hallmark of ECF volume overload is the presence of generalized edema. ECF volume expansion can be associated with proportional increases in the volume of the intravascular and interstitial spaces (e.g., renal failure, nephrotic syndrome, or early hepatic cirrhosis), with maldistribution of fluid across the capillary membrane in which expansion of the interstitial space co-exists with intravascular volume depletion (e.g., capillary leak syndrome or severe hypoalbuminemia), and with effective arterial hypovolemia despite intravascular and interstitial volume expansion (e.g., congestive heart failure). Edema is best noted in dependent portions of the body, such as the lower extremities when standing or the presacral area when supine. Other physical findings of volume expansion are the presence of ascites, jugular venous distension, and signs of left ventricular volume overload (e.g., S_3 gallop and pulmonary edema).

ECF Volume Depletion (Decreased Total Body Sodium)

ECF volume depletion may result from relatively selective loss of intravascular fluid (e.g., hemorrhage or third space sequestration) or from proportional losses of both intravascular and interstitial fluid produced whenever Na intake is less than Na losses. The physical exam, although not a sensitive guide, does provide an estimate of the volume deficit. Volume deficits of less than 10% are compensated for by an increase in vascular resistance and an acceleration in heart rate; thus, except for an increased pulse (which may still be in the normal range), such deficits cannot be easily detected by physical exam. Volume deficits between 10% and 15% cause orthostasis (a decrease in blood pressure and an increase in pulse on assuming an upright position). Deficits between 15% and 25% are associated with a decline in cardiac output and supine hypotension. When volume deficits approach 40%, frank shock occurs. Additional signs of ECF volume contraction include dry mucous membranes, decreased axillary sweat, and skin tenting.

Laboratory findings of Na depletion include prerenal azotemia (BUN/creatinine ratio of $>20:1$) and hyperuricemia. When renal losses are not the cause of the Na depletion, oliguria, low urine sodium (<10 mEq/L) and a concentrated urine are the rule. These laboratory findings indicate decreased renal perfusion and therefore cannot by themselves distinguish absolute volume depletion from effective volume depletion.

DISORDERS OF SODIUM HOMEOSTASIS

ECF Volume Overload

Congestive Heart Failure

A decrease in cardiac output activates neurohormonal effectors designed to restore tissue perfusion. The resultant increase in renal sodium reabsorption expands the volume of the ECF space, increases cardiac preload, and returns cardiac output toward normal at the expense of total body Na overload. With further declines in cardiac output, progressive ventricular dilation and elevated systemic vascular resistance increase myocardial work and thus become maladaptive.

Therapy of congestive heart failure is aimed at improving cardiac output directly by using inotropes (e.g., digoxin) or indirectly by decreasing afterload (vasodilators or ACE inhibitors). Diuretics are a useful adjunct to therapy, but because these agents cause a further decline in effective arterial blood volume, caution is recommended.

Nephrotic Syndrome

Most adults with nephrotic syndrome appear to have a primary inability to excrete Na. Treatment of the volume overload can be accomplished by Na restriction and the judicious use of diuretics. In some patients with nephrotic syndrome, however, intravascular volume depletion secondary to the severe hypoalbuminemia (decreased oncotic pressure) may be present. In these individuals diuretics will further compromise intravascular volume.

Hepatic Cirrhosis

The proximate cause of the Na overload in cirrhosis is controversial. Measurements of intravascular volume are typically elevated in patients with cirrhosis. Increased intrahepatic pressure may stimulate renal Na reabsorption directly or, by causing vasodilation (especially of the splanchnic and mesenteric circulation), secondarily activate renal Na conservation.

A low Na diet and the use of diuretics (spironolactone in particular) are beneficial in the treatment of the Na overload. However, it is important to monitor these patients for signs of intravascular volume depletion.

Renal Failure

Mild degrees of renal insufficiency are not associated with volume overload. As the number of functioning nephrons decline and GFR becomes severely compromised, Na excretion may become limited. Therapy consists of a low Na diet and loop diuretics. When these therapeutic maneuvers are unsuccessful, dialysis should be instituted.

ECF Volume Overload with Intravascular Volume Depletion

Capillary Leak Syndromes

Toxic insults or damage to the capillary endothelium can result in a maldistribution of fluid across the capillary bed. This "capillary leak" can occur with sepsis, secondary to snake bites, or after the administration of certain drugs like interleukin-2. Characteristic of this syndrome is the coexistence of edema and physical findings of intravascular volume depletion. Treatment should be directed at blood pressure support.

Severe Hypoalbuminemia

Although a decrease in oncotic pressure should lead to an increased flux of fluid across the capillary, hypoalbuminemia does not lead to edema unless quite severe (serum albumin <2 g/dL). Redistribution of fluid from the intravascular to the interstitial space in patients with hypoalbuminemia is ameliorated by a variety of countermanding forces, including augmentation of lymphatic return, decrease in interstitial oncotic pressure caused by the washout of interstitial proteins, and increase in interstitial hydrostatic pressure. Thus, unless severe, hypoalbuminemia is not a primary factor in edema formation.

ECF Volume Depletion

Renal Sodium Losses

A urine sodium measurement of greater than 20 mEq/L in the presence of signs of ECF volume contraction indicates renal Na wasting. The most common cause of renal salt wasting is the use of diuretics. The osmotic diuresis induced by hyperglycemia also can be associated with significant renal Na losses. Renal salt wasting occasionally is seen after the relief of urinary obstruction, or in patients with medullary cystic disease.

Extrarenal Sodium Losses

Massive amounts of Na-rich fluid can be lost from the gastrointestinal tract in patients who are vomiting, or who have diarrhea. Significant cutaneous losses of Na-containing fluid can occur in patients with burns, or through strenuous exercise in hot, humid climates. ECF volume depletion also may result from hemorrhage or from the sequestration ("third spacing") of fluid, which can occur in crush injury, intestinal obstruction or infarction, or pancreatitis.

Treatment

The goals of therapy are to prevent ongoing volume losses and to restore ECF volume. Isotonic saline (0.9% NaCl; 154 mEq Na^+/L) is the fluid of choice for volume expansion. The replacement of other electrolytes is best accomplished on an individual basis rather then relying on pre-mixed solutions. The benefits of colloid solutions over crystalloid solutions have not been reliably demonstrated; therefore, considering their cost, the routine use of colloids in fluid resuscitation cannot be recommended.

GENERAL READINGS

Dorhout Mees EJ, Geers AB, Koomans HA: Blood volume and sodium retention in the nephrotic syndrome: a controversial pathophysiological concept. Nephron 36:201, 1984

Dzau VJ: Renal and circulatory mechanisms in congestive heart failure. Kidney Int 31:1402, 1987

Schrier RW: Pathogenesis of sodium and water retention in high-output and low-output cardiac failure, nephrotic syndrome, cirrhosis, and pregnancy. New Engl J Med 319:1065, 1127, 1988

Schrier RW: Body fluid volume regulation in health and disease: a unifying hypothesis. Ann Intern Med 113:155, 1990

CASE STUDY 1

Volume Depletion

Ms. Lucy Bowles, a 25-year-old woman, presented to the hospital complaining of severe diarrhea and mild nausea for five days. Several of her coworkers have had a similar illness. Besides the diarrhea, she also noted increased thirst, fatigue, and a feeling of lightheadedness as if she is going to "pass out" whenever she stands up. She has no significant past medical history and is on no medications except birth control pills.

On physical examination Ms. Bowles is a thin, ill-appearing woman. She is afebrile and when lying down has a blood pressure of 110/80 with a pulse of 96. On standing, her blood pressure is 90/70 with a pulse of 124. She has dry mucous membranes. Her skin turgor appears normal, although her skin is dry. Her neck veins show no engorgement while she is lying flat. There is mild diffuse tenderness on abdominal exam. The rest of her physical exam is unremarkable.

LABORATORY DATA

Na^+ 139 mEq/L	HCO_3 19 mEq/L
K^+ 3.1 mEq/L	BUN 24 mg/dL
Cl^- 110 mEq/L	Creatinine 1.0 mg/dL

Question 1. What is this patient's volume status and what are the physical findings that support your conclusion?

Question 2. Which specific laboratory tests show that this woman is volume depleted?

Question 3. Which other tests may help you decide if the kidney is conserving Na?
Question 4. Explain the mechanisms involved in renal Na retention in this case.
Question 5. How would you treat this patient?

---

1. **What is this patient's volume status and what are the physical findings that support your conclusion?**

Both the history and physical examination provide evidence for volume depletion in this woman. Large quantities of salt and H_2O can be lost from the body during episodes of severe diarrhea. In fact, more than 100,000 people die of diarrhea each year. The Na concentration in severe diarrhea can approach that of plasma. In cases of cholera, volume losses can easily exceed 1 liter each hour. Volume depletion stimulates the release of various dipsogens, leading to increased thirst.[1] Volume depletion also may be associated with a craving for salt (e.g., pizza with anchovies).[2] The complaints of lightheadedness and fatigue occur because of a decrease in cardiac output.

   Physical examination provides confirmatory evidence that the patient is volume depleted. On standing her pulse increases by greater than 20 bpm and her blood pressure decreases. Normally, standing causes the pooling of blood in the lower extremities, a decrease in cardiac preload, and a mild decline in cardiac output. This decline in cardiac output activates compensatory mechanisms designed to prevent falls in perfusion pressure. Heart rate and systemic vascular resistance increase slightly. Thus, after 1 to 2 minutes, if intravascular volume is normal, standing should be associated with a mild increase in heart rate (<10 bpm), an insignificant drop in systolic blood pressure (<10 mmHg) and no change—or even a rise—in diastolic blood pressure. When intravascular volume depletion exceeds 15%, homeostatic mechanisms, already having been activated in the supine position, are no longer able to compensate for the further decline in preload that occurs with standing. Orthostatic hypotension, as defined by an accelerated heart rate (>20 bpm) and a fall in blood pressure (systolic >20 mmHg, diastolic >10 mmHg), becomes evident. Patients with diabetes mellitus, Parkinson's disease, or other forms of autonomic neuropathy, or who are taking a variety of medications (e.g., antihypertensives or tranquilizers) may have these changes without being volume depleted. Further signs of volume depletion in this woman are dry mucous membranes and the lack of detectable jugular venous pressure while lying flat.

2. **Which specific laboratory tests show that this woman is volume depleted?**

The ratio of blood urea nitrogen (BUN) to creatinine (normally 10:1) is one indicator that Ms. Bowles is volume depleted. Both these nitrogenous compounds are freely filtered at the glomerulus and, therefore, as long as their production is fixed, serum concentrations reflect glomerular filtration. However, although there is no tubular reabsorption of creatinine, urea nitrogen does undergo tubular reabsorption. In states of antidiuresis, reabsorption of urea is increased in the distal nephron.[3,4] In Na avid conditions, such as volume depletion, the serum concentration of BUN increases out of proportion to creatinine. In this patient the BUN/creatinine ratio is 24:1, which supports the diagnosis of volume depletion. An elevated BUN/creatinine ratio also can occur if urea production is increased, as occurs with exogenous (protein supplementation) or endogenous (blood in the GI tract, catabolic states) protein loads.

3. Which other tests may help you determine if the kidney is conserving sodium?

The essential sign of renal Na retention is a low urinary Na measurement (<20 mEq/L). The kidney's response to extrarenal volume depletion is to reabsorb Na and H_2O from the urine. Urinary Na concentration can be measured on a spot urine sample. For diagnostic accuracy, this should be obtained before beginning any volume repletion therapy. Partial treatment of volume depletion decreases the stimulus for the kidney to hold onto Na and the urinary Na may be greater than 20 mEq/L. When volume depletion results from vomiting, the kidney dumps bicarbonate in an effort to correct the concomitant alkalosis. The bicarbonate pulls Na along with it.[5] Thus, urinary sodium may be abnormally elevated despite extrarenal Na depletion. In this situation, a low urinary chloride is a better indicator of volume depletion. If the cause of the volume depletion is renal Na wasting (as occurs with diuretics, osmotic loads, or occasionally with renal diseases such as medullary cystic disease) the urinary Na and Cl are both elevated.

4. Explain the mechanisms involved in renal sodium retention in this case.

Intravascular volume contraction results in decreased preload with subsequent fall in cardiac output, blood pressure and renal perfusion (Fig. 1-3). Baroreceptors in the aortic arch and carotids sense the fall in blood pressure and by means of a CNS processor increase sympathetic output. The increase in renal sympathetic activity, along with decreased perfusion pressure, stimulates renin release. Renin promotes the production of AII. AII directly increases reabsorp-

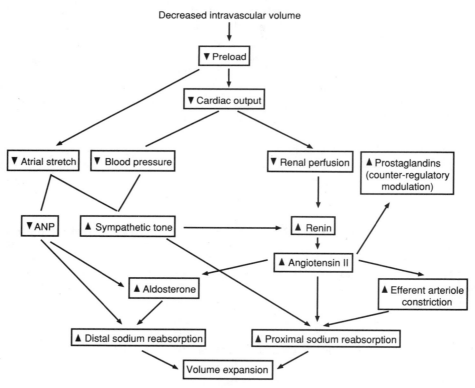

Fig. 1-3. Summary of the physiologic events leading to the correction of intravascular volume depletion.

tion of Na in the proximal tubule by activating Na-H exchange,[6] and indirectly increases it by selectively constricting the efferent glomerular arteriole,[7,8] which increases the fraction of plasma filtered at the glomerulus, and thus raises the oncotic pressure in the peritubular capillaries. AII also stimulates aldosterone release. Aldosterone enhances Na reabsorption in the distal tubule. In addition, because of decreased atrial stretch, atrial natriuretic peptide release is inhibited, further promoting renal Na reabsorption.

5. How would you treat this patient?

By the time orthostatic hypotension appears, ECF volume has contracted by at least 15% or approximately 30 mL/kg. The aim of therapy is to replace the volume losses until the patient is normovolemic. Because the patient is orthostatic, oral therapy alone is inadequate. Intravenous fluids should be started. Volume depletion should be treated with isotonic saline (154 mEq/L) which is confined exclusively to the ECF space. The use of more hypotonic fluids is to be avoided because of their greater volume of distribution. If other electrolyte abnormalities are present (such as hypokalemia in this case), fluids that are individually tailored to the situation should be used rather than premixed solutions (e.g., Ringer's lactate). Volume depletion secondary to blood loss should be treated with packed red cells. Although it could be argued that intravascular volume depletion should be treated with colloid solutions (e.g., albumin or plasmanate) that remain within the vasculature instead of distributing throughout the entire ECF space, the lack of clear benefit of these solutions[9,10] along with their prohibitive cost makes their use unwarranted.

Enough isotonic saline should be administered to reverse any hemodynamic compromise present. In a young healthy individual like Ms. Bowles several liters of saline can be rapidly infused until orthostasis is relieved. In patients with renal insufficiency or heart failure, overly zealous fluid resuscitation can result in pulmonary edema. In such patients, treatment should consist of isotonic saline boluses (250 to 500 mL). After each bolus, the patient's volume status needs to be reevaluated. After intravascular volume has been repleted, fluid replacement should equal the rate of fluid loss.

CASE STUDY 2

Volume Overload Associated with Congestive Heart Failure

Mr. Al Corona, a 60-year-old man, was admitted to the hospital complaining of worsening shortness of breath, which has increased during the past 2 weeks. He has also noticed so much swelling in his lower extremities that it is difficult to put on his shoes.

Past medical history is significant for cardiovascular disease. Over the past 10 years the patient has had several "heart attacks," which have left him with a "damaged heart." He is presently taking digoxin, furosemide, and an unknown pain medication recently prescribed for back pain. The patient denies using excessive salt. However, Mr. Corona has been eating more canned and prepackaged foods lately since his wife is away visiting relatives.

On physical exam the patient appears in moderate respiratory distress. His blood pressure is 160/100 with an irregular pulse rate of 136. Respiratory rate is 28. Jugular venous pressure is 11 cm. On cardiac exam the point of maximum impulse is diffuse and laterally displaced. There is a II/VI holosystolic murmur at the apex that radiates to the axilla. A soft S_3 is audible. Rales are present at both lung bases. Edema to the midtibia is present bilaterally.

LABORATORY DATA

Na^+ 130 mEq/L	HCO_3^- 29 mEq/L	Urinary Na^+ 8 mEq/L
K^+ 3.5 mEq/L	BUN 50 mg/dL	
Cl^- 92 mEq/L	Creatine 2.0 mg/dL	

EKG: atrial fibrillation with ventricular response of approximately 130 bpm; Q waves in V_{1-3} and poor R wave progression.

Chest X-ray: cardiomegaly and bilateral infiltrates in the lower lobes consistent with congestive heart failure and mild pulmonary edema.

Question 1. Can you determine the patient's volume status from the clinical description?

Question 2. Although Mr. Corona exhibits obvious signs and symptoms of total body Na overload, he is retaining Na. Why?

Question 3. Explain the role of each of the following systems in the pathophysiology of Na retention by the kidney:
   a. renin-angiotensin-aldosterone system
   b. sympathetic nervous system
   c. peritubular capillary forces
   d. vasopressin
   e. atrial natriuretic hormone

Question 4. The medication for Mr. Corona's back pain was found to be indomethacin, a prostaglandin synthesis inhibitor. The patient had been taking this medication every 6 hours for the past week. How could this have contributed to the patient's present state of Na retention and his increased BUN and creatinine over baseline?

Question 5. Describe nonpharmacologic interventions that could help treat this patient.

Question 6. The patient requires pharmacologic therapy to become comfortable. Which medications may be beneficial?

Question 7. Despite appropriate medical management, the patient develops oliguria and increasing renal insufficiency. You have stopped all possible offending agents, but the patient is becoming hypoxic from pulmonary edema. What other medicine may help in an intensive care setting?

---

1. Can you determine the patient's volume status from the clinical description?

Symptoms and physical findings clearly indicate total body Na overload. Both the intravascular space, as demonstrated by the elevated jugular venous pressure, and the interstitial space, as confirmed by the peripheral edema and rales on lung exam, are expanded. The presence of an audible S_3 indicates ventricular volume overload. The chest radiograph reveals evidence of pulmonary vascular congestion, corroborating the physical findings. Renal Na retention has resulted in an increase in intravascular volume and pressure with subsequent movement of salt and water into the interstitial space.

2. Although Mr. Corona exhibits obvious signs and symptoms of total body Na overload, he is retaining Na. Why?

As the pumping function of the heart deteriorates, the normal relationship between stroke volume and left ventricular end-diastolic volume shifts downward. Less stroke volume, and therefore less cardiac output, is achieved for a given end-diastolic volume. This fall in cardiac output activates neurohormonal mechanisms that produce vasoconstriction and antinatriuresis. The subsequent expansion of the intravascular fluid space improves cardiac output by increasing end-diastolic volume and stroke volume. Thus, cardiac output is maintained at the expense of engorgement of the ECF space. Upon normalization of the cardiac output, Na excretion again equals sodium intake and a new steady state is achieved. A further decline in cardiac output reactivates these vasoconstrictive and antinatriuretic processes. Although initially beneficial, these processes (systemic vascular resistance and ventricular wall tension) can become counterproductive by increasing afterload,[11] actually increasing the work of the heart and causing further declines in cardiac output.

3. Explain the role of each of the following systems in the pathophysiology of Na retention by the kidney:
    a. renin-angiotensin-aldosterone system
    b. sympathetic nervous system
    c. peritubular capillary forces
    d. vasopressin
    e. atrial natriuretic hormone

a. Renin-angiotensin-aldosterone system

A poorly functioning heart is unable to pump blood adequately to the peripheral tissues. The decrease in blood flow to the afferent glomerular arteriole stimulates renin secretion, which converts angiotensinogen to angiotensin I. Angiotensin converting enzyme (ACE) cleaves angiotensin I to angiotensin II, a potent vasoconstrictor. Within the kidney, AII selectively constricts the efferent arteriole, increasing the fraction of plasma filtered at the glomerulus and maintaining GFR despite lower renal blood flow.[7,8] The increase in filtration fraction by elevating peritubular capillary oncotic pressure favors the reabsorption of Na and H_2O. Angiotensin II activation of the Na/H antiporter in the proximal tubule also increases sodium reabsorption.[6] In addition, AII stimulates aldosterone secretion, which in turn facilitates sodium reabsorption by the distal tubule. Finally, AII stimulates intrarenal prostaglandin synthesis.[12] Prostaglandins appear to serve a counter-regulatory function.[12]

b. Sympathetic nervous system

The activity of the sympathetic nervous system in congestive heart failure is modulated by two conflicting occurrences: decreased cardiac output and atrial distention. Because plasma and urinary catecholamine levels are elevated in CHF,[13] the fall in blood pressure and tissue perfusion appears to take precedence over venous congestion. Whether the CNS processor has developed to prioritize blood pressure or whether the overall response is an integration of these two contradictory inputs is unclear. The rise in plasma catecholamines attenuates the decline in cardiac output by increasing both heart rate and contractility. Catecholamines and AII cause arteriolar constriction in attempts to maintain blood pressure and tissue perfusion.

c. Peritubular capillary forces

Sodium reabsorption in the proximal tubule is regulated by the physical forces that exist in the pericapillary tubules and the interstitium. The difference in oncotic pressure and hydrostatic pressure between these two compartments determines whether salt and H_2O move from the interstitium into the capillary network or backleak into the tubular lumen.[14,15] Pressure for reabsorption = $f[(\pi_c - \pi_i) - (P_c - P_i)]$, where f = a constant, π = oncotic pressure, P = hydrostatic pressure, c = peritubular capillary, and i = interstitium. In a low flow state like congestive heart failure, the selective constriction of the efferent arteriole by AII increases the fraction of plasma filtered at the glomerulus, thus maintaining a constant GFR despite reduced renal plasma flow. Constriction of the efferent arteriole results in a decrease in hydrostatic pressure and a rise in oncotic pressure in the peritubular capillaries that arise from the efferent arteriole. These changes in physical factors favor the movement of salt and H_2O from the lateral intercellular space into the peritubular capillary.

d. Arginine vasopressin (anti-diuretic hormone)

A decline in effective arterial volume serves as a nonosmotic stimulus to vasopressin secretion. In addition to being a vasoconstrictor, vasopressin, by facilitating the reabsorption of H_2O by the kidney, expands volume at the expense of tonicity. The presence of hyponatremia in CHF, as seen in this patient, implies elevated ADH level and is indicative of cardiac decompensation and poor prognosis.[16]

e. Atrial natriuretic peptide

Atrial distention results in ANP release. This peptide causes an increase in renal vasodilatation and natriuresis. Although ANP levels are elevated in chronic CHF, antinatriuresis predominates, suggesting that the renal response to ANP may be blunted in chronic heart failure.[17-19] In all likelihood, ANP functions as a counter-regulatory modulator. Blocking ANP action exacerbates Na retention and volume overload in CHF.[19] Further increasing ANP levels in CHF by infusing pharmacologic doses or by inhibiting its degradation causes vasodilation and natriuresis.[17,18,20]

4.   **You discover that the medication for Mr. Corona's back pain was indomethacin, a prostaglandin synthesis inhibitor. The patient has been taking this medication every 6 hours for the past week. How could this have contributed to the patient's present state of Na retention and his increased BUN and creatinine over baseline?**

Nonsteroidal anti-inflammatory drugs (NSAIDs) inhibit prostaglandin synthesis. Renal vasodilatory prostaglandins are stimulated by AII to counteract renal vasoconstriction and to promote salt and H_2O excretion. Renal perfusion is thus maintained despite systemic vasoconstriction. In addition, the vasodilatory prostaglandins help to diminish the magnitude of the antinatriuretic response. By inhibiting normal prostaglandin synthesis, acute renal failure may result from a decrease in renal perfusion. Furthermore, by blocking prostaglandin synthesis, Na retention becomes unopposed, which results in worsening volume overload. NSAIDs, therefore, should be used with caution in individuals with diminished cardiac reserve.[21]

5. Describe nonpharmacologic interventions that could help treat this patient.

Two nonpharmacologic treatments helpful in the treatment of CHF are dietary salt restriction and bedrest. Bedrest decreases sympathetic activity and produces a fall in plasma catecholamine levels. The subsequent decline in systemic vascular resistance reduces the impedance against which the heart must pump and improves cardiac output. In addition, a horizontal position favors reabsorption of interstitial fluid from the lower extremities, thereby increasing central venous return to the heart and further improving stroke volume. Bedrest has been shown to cause a 40% increase in GFR and a doubling of natriuresis in response to diuretics. Sodium restriction is another important adjuvant therapy in the treatment of CHF. The normal American diet contains approximately 10 to 12 g NaCl (salt) a day (4–4.8 g Na^+). The canned and prepackaged foods Mr. Aloni had been eating frequently are high in Na and can cause worsening Na overload. For severe congestive heart failure, salt intake should be limited to approximately 4 g/day (≈ 1.6 g Na^+), which is equivalent to a no-added salt diet (no salt used for cooking or flavoring). More severe Na restriction is difficult to maintain outside a hospital setting and often leads to noncompliance. The intake of fluid should be restricted to 2 L/day. More stringent restriction may be necessary if hyponatremia exists.

6. The patient requires pharmacologic therapy to become comfortable. Which medications may be beneficial?

Three types of medications that may be effective in treating this patient are diuretics, digitalis glycosides, and an angiotensin-converting-enzyme inhibitor. These medications counter the maladaptive mechanisms that contribute to his symptoms.

Diuretics inhibit renal Na reabsorption, promote natriuresis, and decrease ECF volume. The decrease in intravascular volume reduces intravascular pressure, and excess fluid moves out of the lungs and periphery, providing symptomatic relief. The decrease in plasma volume also results in a fall in cardiac preload, a reduction in the size of the left ventricular cavity, and a decline in wall tension. The overall effect of these hemodynamic changes on ventricular performance may be positive or negative depending upon where along the Frank-Starling curve the myocardium is functioning. The decrease in wall tension (a component of afterload) improves fiber shortening, but the decline in preload may have the opposite effect if the heart is on the ascending part of the curve. Excessive diuresis can lead to a fall in cardiac output. In severe heart failure it is often necessary to accept a decline in cardiac output to improve symptoms.

Digitalis glycosides are not only direct cardiac inotropes, but by slowing the ventricular response they also allow more time for adequate ventricular filling. These drugs cause a rise in intracellular sodium by inhibiting Na^+, K^+-ATPase. Sodium exits the cell in exchange for calcium. The subsequent elevation in intracellular Ca enhances contractility. The effect of the digitalis glycosides on atrioventricular conduction is secondary to increases in vagal tone.[22]

ACE inhibitors are rapidly becoming the mainstay of therapy for congestive heart failure. The inhibition of angiotensin-converting enzyme reduces the conversion of AI to AII, resulting in renal and systemic vasodilatation. The decrease in blood pressure reduces the load against which the heart must pump, thereby decreasing myocardial work and improving cardiac output. Unlike diuretics, these agents can prevent progressive cardiac dysfunction.[23-25] Patients with severe heart failure (New York Heart Association class III) who are treated with an ACE inhibitor have a decrease in cardiovascular mortality compared to patients not treated with this medication.[23-25] ACE inhibitors selectively increase renal blood flow. In animal studies of congestive heart failure, renal blood flow and single-nephron GFR increase secondary to decreased efferent arteriolar resistance. Patients with CHF treated with ACE inhibitors show improvement in renal function and decreased diuretic requirements.[26]

Side effects of ACE inhibitor therapy include hypotension and a decline in renal function. If arterial vasodilation is not accompanied by an adequate increase in cardiac output, blood pressure and renal perfusion will decline. This commonly occurs as an effect secondary to excessive preload reduction from overdiuresis. A decrease in diuretic dosage often reverses these side effects. Renal function may also deteriorate in the presence of bilateral renal artery stenosis. With decreased renal perfusion, GFR is preserved by the constriction of the efferent arteriole. Inhibiting angiotensin II causes efferent arteriole vasodilatation. Because of the fixed stenoses, renal perfusion can not increase and GFR falls.

Mr. Corona must be treated carefully because of his baseline renal insufficiency. He has known cardiovascular disease and a possibility of severe renovascular disease exists. Captopril, a short-acting ACE inhibitor, can be initiated at a low dose (6.25 mg) and titrated upward if there are no deleterious effects on either blood pressure or renal function. If the patient fails ACE inhibitor therapy, nitrates (preload reduction), and hydralazine, a direct arterial vasodilator (afterload reduction), may be tried in combination.

7. **Despite appropriate medical management, the patient develops oliguria and increasing renal insufficiency. All possible offending agents have been stopped, but the patient is becoming hypoxic from pulmonary edema. What other medicine may help in an intensive care setting?**

Low-dose dopamine, by binding to dopaminergic receptors within the vasculature and the kidney, increases renal blood flow and directly inhibits Na reabsorption in the proximal tubule.[27,28] Furthermore, dopamine at doses between 2 and 5 µg/kg/m activates β-adrenergic receptors, increasing cardiac contractility. This combination of events makes dopamine an ideal agent to use in refractory heart failure.

CASE STUDY 3

Cirrhosis and Ascites

Mr. Bob Daniels, a 50-year-old man, presented to the hospital complaining of increasing abdominal girth. He has a long history of alcohol abuse. Several years ago he had been admitted to the hospital for treatment of gastritis. At that time he was told he had a "fatty liver" caused by his alcohol consumption. He says that he has noticed progressive distention of his abdomen over the past year, despite having a poor appetite and minimal weight gain. He admits to drinking approximately one pint of whiskey a day. Two months ago he was told that his eyes appeared yellow. Lately, he has also noted occasional episodes of shortness of breath, especially when lying flat.

Other than the previous admission, his past medical history is unremarkable. He has not seen a physician for the past 3 years and takes no medications.

On physical exam, Mr. Daniels is a lethargic man who appears to be chronically ill, with a protuberant abdomen. He is afebrile. Blood pressure is 98/50 mmHg with no orthostatic changes. Pulse is 100. Respiratory rate is 24 breaths/m. He is markedly icteric and has multiple spider telangiectasias on his arms, thorax, and upper back. Decreased breath sounds are present at both bases. Gynecomastia is present. Abdominal exam reveals a protuberant abdomen with an easily demonstrable fluid wave. The liver edge is not palpable. He has guaiac-positive brown stool. His lower extremities exhibit trace edema. Asterixis is present.

LABORATORY DATA

Na^+ 133 mEq/L	Creatinine 1.0 mg/dL	PT 16 seconds (1.4 times control)
K^+ 3.4 mEq/L	Total bilirubin 7.0	PTT 29 seconds
Cl^- 106 mEq/L	AST 140	Hct 32%
HCO_3^- 18 mEq/L	ALT of 80	Platelet count 76,000
BUN 8 mg/dL	Albumin 2.6 gm/dL	

Question 1. Based on the history and physical how would you characterize Mr. Daniel's volume status?

Question 2. Are there laboratory tests that may be helpful in ascertaining the "fullness" of Mr. Daniel's circulation?

Question 3. What are the proposed pathophysiologic mechanisms responsible for sodium retention in liver disease?

Question 4. What nonpharmacologic therapy would you offer this patient? What pharmacologic intervention would you use if these measures failed?

---

1. Based on the history and physical how would you characterize Mr. Daniel's volume?

Both the history of progressive abdominal distension and physical exam findings of ascites and lower extremity edema point to ECF overload. Edema typically cannot be identified on physical exam until the interstitial space has been expanded by approximately 5 liters. The amount of ascites necessary before physical findings (i.e., bulging flanks, shifting dullness, fluid wave) become apparent is unknown, but in this patient who has obvious abdominal distension, an additional 5 liters of fluid are likely present within his abdomen. Thus, Mr. Daniel's ECF space is expanded by at least 10 liters. The status of this patient's intravascular space is less clear. Physical examination reveals a BP of 98/50. Although this is low, orthostatic changes are not present, which suggests that the intravascular space is not significantly depleted. The low BP and wide pulse pressure are probably caused by systemic vasodilation and opening of arteriovenous shunts secondary to the underlying liver disease.

2. Are there laboratory tests that may be helpful in ascertaining the "fullness" of Mr. Daniel's intravascular space?

The volume of the intravascular space can be quantified isotopically with radiolabeled albumin or by dye dilution techniques that use dyes confined to the intravascular space (i.e., Evans blue). These techniques provide reliable estimates of plasma volume, but do not necessarily reflect circulatory fullness. For example, vasodilation of the arterial circulation will decrease effective arterial blood volume despite having little or no effect on intravascular volume. Similarly, congestive heart failure is associated with decreased effective volume even though the intravascular space is expanded. Thus, although quantifying the volume of the intravascular space is useful for research purposes, it provides little clinical information.

The adequacy of the circulation can be indirectly assessed by measuring the concentration of hormonal effectors of Na and volume homeostasis. Elevated levels of renin, aldosterone, angiotensin, ADH, and plasma catecholamines would suggest that there is underfilling of the circulation with stimulation of vasoconstrictive and antinatriuretic hormones. The clinical utility of these measurements, however, is unclear.

Another means of assessing the effectiveness of the arterial circulation is by measuring urinary Na. Because the kidneys, if normal, are the ultimate mediators of Na balance, urinary Na excretion reflects the adequacy of the circulation. A low urinary Na usually indicates an inadequate vascular volume and secondary stimulation of renal Na retention.

3. What are the proposed pathophysiologic mechanisms responsible for sodium retention in liver disease?

The pathophysiology of Na retention in chronic liver disease has not been completely resolved. Two competing theories have been proposed: the classical underfilling theory and the overflow theory. According to advocates of underfilling, portal hypertension and hypoalbuminemia lead to the transudation of fluid out of the hepatic sinusoids, overwhelming the ability of the hepatic lymphatics to return it to the circulation. This excess fluid escapes, freely weeping from the liver capsule into the peritoneum. The underfill theory presumes that renal Na retention is secondary to the loss of extracellular fluid into the peritoneum as ascites.

The fact that central blood volume expansion produced by head-out water immersion is often natriuretic in patients with cirrhosis supports the role of vascular underfilling in the etiology of Na retention in this disease.[29] Further support comes from studies that have demonstrated increased levels of circulating antinatriuretic hormones in Na-retentive cirrhotic patients.[30,31]

There are, however, several criticisms of the underfill theory. Plasma volume when measured has been found to be expanded in patients with cirrhosis and ascites compared to normal patients.[32,33] Furthermore, in several animal models Na retention actually precedes ascites formation.[34,35] Prevention of ascites by creation of an end-to-side portacaval shunt does not reduce the Na retention.[36] However, amelioration of intrahepatic hypertension with a side-to-side portal caval shunt does decrease renal Na reabsorption.[34] The overflow theory postulates that the primary cause for the formation of ascites is renal sodium retention. Intrahepatic hypertension results in intense Na avidity, possibly through increased renal sympathetic activity. The subsequent expansion of plasma volume leads secondarily to ascites.

The overflow theory of ascites formation cannot account for the elevated concentration of neurohormonal mediators found in some patients with ascites and liver disease. A unifying hypothesis recently has been advanced.[37] This hypothesis proposes that intrahepatic hypertension leads to vasodilation and to opening of portal-systemic and arteriovenous shunts. Such a theory would explain the decreased systemic vascular resistance, activation of antinatriuretic and vasoconstrictive hormones, renal Na retention, and expanded plasma volume commonly present in cirrhosis.

4. What nonpharmacologic therapy would you offer this patient? What pharmacologic intervention would you use if these measures failed?

Ascites is more then just a cosmetic inconvenience. It can lead to decreased nutritional intake, compromised cardiac output, and, most importantly, bacterial peritonitis. Thus, in most circumstances treatment should be initiated. The simplest therapy for ascites and edema is Na restriction and bedrest. Salt intake should be limited to less than 500 mg/day. This can be liberalized to 1 g/d if the patient is improving. Fluid intake also should be minimized, especially in the face of hyponatremia. Bedrest decreases catecholamine levels and increases intravascular volume (by decreasing the gravitational forces responsible for dependent edema). It also maximizes renal perfusion and Na excretion. Although safe and efficacious, such therapy is time consuming and not in keeping with modern medical practice.

More rapid mobilization of ascitic fluid can be accomplished using diuretics or high-volume paracentesis. No matter which method is chosen, ascites will reaccumulate unless Na restriction is also instituted. Absorption of fluid from the peritoneum into the vasculature is limited.[38] Therefore, in the absence of edema, diuresis should be restricted to approximately 500 to 750 mL/d. Excessive diuresis can cause intravascular volume depletion and renal failure. Because interstitial fluid is more easily mobilized than ascitic fluid, in the presence of edema, diuresis can be increased to 1,000 to 1,500 mL/d without compromising intravascular volume.

In contrast to other Na-avid conditions, patients with cirrhosis may respond better to spironolactone,[39] an aldosterone antagonist, rather than a loop diuretic like furosemide. Most diuretics are active only from within the tubular lumen. Because of protein binding, diuretics enter the urinary space by tubular secretion rather than glomerular filtration. In patients with liver disease, decreased secretion of diuretics into the tubule occurs, possibly because of the accumulation of bile salts, which may interfere with tubular secretion of the diuretics.[40] Hypoalbuminemia also decreases the amount of diuretic that is delivered to the tubular lumen.[41] Spironolactone, however, does not require tubular secretion for diuretic activity; it freely passes from the plasma into the cell where it binds to the aldosterone receptor. The inhibition of aldosterone reduces Na reabsorption in the cortical collecting duct. Another advantage of this diuretic is that it does not cause K depletion, which, by increasing ammoniagenesis, can exacerbate hepatic encephalopathy. Because of the potential for hyperkalemia, K monitoring is extremely important. In patients with a tendency toward hyperkalemia (e.g., diabetics, renal failure patients), spironolactone should be avoided.

Large volume paracentesis has also been shown to be efficacious and safe for the treatment of ascites.[42] Removal of 3 to 5 liters of ascitic fluid is usually well tolerated. Concerns that such treatment might result in rapid reaccumulation of peritoneal fluid with intravascular compromise has led to the recommendation that albumin infusions be used with this technique. Whether this is necessary is unclear. If the patient has a baseline low blood pressure and greater than 3 liters of ascites are to be removed, albumin may be beneficial.

CASE STUDY 4

Nephrotic Syndrome

Mr. Tamm Horsfall is a 32-year-old white man referred to you because of complaints of swelling in his arms, legs, and around his eyes. The swelling has progressed over the last month or two. He denies history of heart disease or chest pain. He has not had any episodes of fever, chills, or weight loss. On further questioning he states that he has noticed that his urine has been exceedingly foamy for the past month. Several weeks ago, his private doctor started him on furosemide 20 mg per day for some ankle swelling. This medication initially caused him to urinate more, but has not helped the swelling. He returned to his local physician for routine follow-up and was referred to you for evaluation.

His past medical history is unremarkable. He has no history of intravenous drug abuse and denies participating in any activities associated with a risk of HIV infection. He occasionally takes ibuprofen for some back pain, but takes no other medications.

On physical examination the patient is grossly edematous, especially periorbitally. He is afebrile; blood pressure is 165/100 mmHg (without orthostasis) with a heart rate of 104 beats/m, and respiratory rate of 16 breaths/m. His cardiac exam is unremarkable except for elevated neck veins. Chest exam reveals decreased breath sounds at the bases of both lung fields. Abdominal exam reveals shifting dullness and a fluid wave. The abdominal wall is edematous. There is 4+ pitting edema to the hips.

LABORATORY STUDIES

Na^+ 135 mEq/L	BUN 18 mg/dL	ALT 30
K^+ 3.8 mEq/L	Creatinine 1.4 mg/dL	Albumin 2.6 g/dL
Cl^- 105 mEq/L	Total bilirubin 1.0	Cholesterol 330 mg/dL
HCO_3^- 24 mEq/L	AST 40	

Urinalysis: 4+ protein, no blood; microscopic: oval fat bodies
24 hour urine protein: 6.7 g
Chest x-ray: Small bilateral pleural effusions. Heart normal size

---

Question 1. What is Mr. Horsfall's diagnosis?
Question 2. What is Mr. Horsfall's volume status?
Question 3. If Starling forces determine the flux of fluid across the capillary bed, why does hypoalbuminemia not cause expansion of the interstitial space?
Question 4. What is the pathophysiology of edema formation in nephrotic syndrome?
Question 4. How would you treat this patient?
Question 5. What diagnostic workup should be pursued in this patient?

---

1. What is Mr. Horsfall's diagnosis?

Mr. Horsfall has nephrotic syndrome. This entity is defined by proteinuria (>3.5 g/24 h), hypoalbuminemia, hyperlipidemia, and edema. Primary glomerular diseases, medications (e.g., penicillamine, captopril, and NSAIDs), infections (e.g., hepatitis B, syphilis, and malaria), and systemic diseases such as diabetes, amyloidosis, cancer, sickle cell anemia, and lupus can cause the nephrotic syndrome.

2. What is Mr. Horsfall's volume status?

This patient clearly has an overload of total body sodium. Both the interstitial space (diffuse edema) and the intravascular space (hypertension and distended neck veins) are expanded. Typical of the volume overload associated with nephrotic syndrome is the lack of left-sided congestive heart failure. In the absence of primary cardiac disease, pulmonary edema is an unusual manifestation of nephrotic syndrome.

3. What is the pathophysiology of edema formation in nephrotic syndrome?

In contrast to congestive heart failure and cirrhosis, in which the kidneys are structurally normal, the nephrotic syndrome is characterized by primary renal damage and decreased renal function in some patients. As with cirrhosis, there are two theories for edema formation: the underfilling theory and the overflow theory. Normally, the urine contains a small amount of protein, usually less than 150 mg/day. This consists primarily of small molecular weight proteins that are secreted into the kidney tubule. Large proteins like albumin are kept out of the urine by the glomerulus, which forms both a size and a charge barrier. In the nephrotic syndrome, glomerular damage alters permeability. Large quantities of protein are filtered at the glomerulus and either metabolized by the tubules or lost in the urine. Hypoalbuminemia results if the liver cannot compensate for urinary protein losses. This is in contrast to cirrhosis in which hypoalbuminemia is a result of decreased hepatic synthesis.

According to the underfill theory, the decrease in plasma oncotic pressure caused by hypoalbuminemia results in transudation of fluid out of the vasculature into the interstitial space. This decrease in plasma volume leads to activation of the sympathetic nervous system and the renin-angiotensin-aldosterone axis. Thus, the kidney retains Na and H_2O as a secondary response to the hypovolemia. Confirmation of this theory is obtained in some nephrotic patients, in particular those with minimal change disease, in whom plasma volume is low, levels of antinatriuretic hormones are elevated, and diuresis often results in signs and symptoms of hypovolemia.[43,44]

Many patients with nephrotic syndrome, however, are hypertensive and have expanded plasma volumes.[45] In addition, the degree of hypoalbuminemia does not correlate with the extent of edema. It is not unusual for a patient with an albumin of 2 g/dL to have minimal or no edema, while a patient with an albumin of 3.4 g/dL may have marked anasarca. Additional criticism of the role of decreased oncotic pressure as a cause of hypovolemia comes from human and animal studies that demonstrate that hypoalbuminemia induced by plasmapheresis does not cause intravascular volume depletion.[46]

If Na retention is not secondary to real or perceived volume depletion, it must be caused by a primary disorder of renal Na excretion. Animal studies of nephrosis experimentally induced by infusing an aminonucleoside into one kidney support the role of primary renal Na retention in nephrotic syndrome.[47] This model produces unilateral proteinuria. Interestingly, in these experiments only the treated kidney retained Na. If volume depletion were the cause of the Na retention, both kidneys should have been sodium avid. Thus, at least in this model, salt retention presumedly is due to a primary abnormality in Na excretion rather than to a secondary response to decreased intravascular volume.

3. If Starling forces determine the flux of fluid across the capillary bed, why does hypoalbuminemia not cause an expansion of the interstitial space?

Although Starling forces do determine the rate of fluid flux across the capillary membrane, there are several countermanding forces that prevent the loss of intravascular fluid into the interstitium. Interstitial hydrostatic pressure is subatmospheric.[48] Increased fluid within the interstitium raises hydrostatic pressure and counters further fluid movement.[48] In addition, the lymphatic flow can accelerate significantly, returning any excess fluid to the vasculature.[49] This increase in fluid movement into the lymphatics washes proteins out of the interstitium and thus decreases interstitial oncotic pressure, further protecting the interstitial space from volume overload.[49,50]

4. How would you treat this patient?

Edema is caused by salt and H_2O retention. Therefore, dietary salt (NaCl) intake should be limited to between 2 and 3 g/day. Natriuresis can be enhanced by maximizing venous return to the heart by prescribing bedrest, elevation of the lower extremities, and the application of pressure stockings to the legs. If these measures are unsuccessful, initiation of diuretic therapy may be beneficial. Patients with nephrotic syndrome, however, may exhibit diuretic resistance. Binding of the diuretic to albumin within the tubular lumen may render the drug inactive.[51] Furthermore, protein binding of a diuretic may be necessary for delivery of the drug to the kidney for secretion.[41] Administration of loop diuretics with albumin has been shown to increase diuresis and improve edema in some diuretic-resistant patients.[41]

If Mr. Horsfall become refractory to high-dose loop diuretics, then a combination of a loop and a thiazide diuretic might be effective.[52] Because inhibition of sodium reabsorption at one nephron site may lead to compensatory increases in sodium reabsorption at other sites, the sequential blockade of the loop of Henle and the distal tubule frequently produces a natriuresis in resistant patients. Complications of this therapy are volume depletion and hypokalemia. Patients in whom combination diuretic therapy is used therefore require close monitoring.

5. What diagnostic workup should be pursued in this patient?

The main categories for nephrotic syndrome discussed above should be used as a differential diagnosis and basis for workup. All possible medications that cause the nephrotic syndrome should be stopped. A serum test for syphilis and hepatitis B surface antigen should be done. Systemic diseases are considered based on history and physical exam. Because nephrotic syndrome may be the presenting manifestation of systemic lupus, complement levels and an ANA are mandatory. Although multiple myeloma is unlikely in this patient, a serum protein electrophoresis and a urine immunoelectrophoresis would be necessary to rule out this disease.

The etiology of the nephrotic syndrome in this patient is not obvious. Ibuprofen is a possible cause. History and physical exam indicate that Mr. Horsfall does not have an obvious systemic disease or infection. If the various blood tests suggested above do not establish a diagnosis, the patient may have an idiopathic glomerulopathy. Such a diagnosis can be made only by a renal biopsy.

REFERENCES

1. Fitzsimons JT: The physiologic basis of thirst. Kidney Int 10:3, 1976
2. Denton DA: The brain and sodium homeostasis conditions. Reflex 8:125, 1973
3. Chasis H, Smith WH: The excretion of urea in normal man and in subjects with glomerulonephritis. J Clin Invest 17:347, 1938
4. Sands JM, Nonoguchi H, Knepper MA: Vasopressin effects on urea and H_2O transport in inner medullary collecting duct subsegments. Am J Physiol 253:F823, 1987
5. Kassirer JP, Schwartz WB: The response of normal man to selective depletion of hydrochloric acid. Am J Med 40:10, 1966
6. Cogan MG: Angiotensin II: a powerful controller of sodium transport in the early proximal tubule. Hypertension 5:451, 1990
7. Ichikawa I, Brenner BM: Importance of efferent arteriolar vascular tone in regulation of proximal tubule fluid reabsorption and glomerulotubular balance in the rat. J Clin Invest 65:1192, 1980
8. Edwards RM: Segmental effects of norepinephrine and angiotensin II on isolated renal microvessels. Am J Physiol 244:F526, 1983

9. Virgilio RW, Rice CL, Smith DE et al: Crystalloid vs colloid resuscitation: is one better? Surgery 85: 129, 1979
10. Erstad BL, Gales BJ, Rappaport WD: The use of albumin in clinical practice. Arch Intern Med 151: 901, 1991
11. Dzau VJ: Renal and circulatory mechanisms in congestive heart failure. Kidney Int 31:1402, 1987
12. Dunn MJ, Scharschmide LA: Prostaglandins modulate the glomerular actions of angiotensin II. Kidney Int 31:S-95–S-101, 1987
13. Thomas JA, Marks BH: Plasma norepinephrine in congestive heart failure. Am J Card 41:233, 1978
14. Brenner BM, Troy JL: Postglomerular vascular protein concentration: evidence for a causal role in governing fluid reabsorption and glomerulotubular balance by the renal proximal tubule. J Clin Invest 50:336, 1971
15. Ichikawa I, Brenner BM: Mechanism of inhibition of proximal tubule fluid reabsorption after exposure of the rat kidney to the physical effects of expansion of extracellular fluid volume. J Clin Invest 64: 1466, 1979
16. Lee WH, Packer M: Prognostic importance of serum sodium concentration and its modification by converting-enzyme inhibition in patients with severe chronic heart failure. Circulation 73:257, 1986
17. Cody RJ, Atlas SA, Laragh JH et al: Atrial natriuretic factor in normal subjects and heart failure patients. J Clin Invest 78:1362, 1986
18. Koepke JP, DiBona GF: Blunted natriuresis to atrial natriuretic peptide in chronic sodium-retaining disorders. Am J Physiol 252:F865, 1987
19. Awazu M, Imada T, Kon V et al: Role of endogenous atrial natriuretic peptide in congestive heart failure. Am J Physiol 257:R641, 1989
20. Perrella MA, Margulies KB, Burnett JC: Pathophysiology of congestive heart failure: role of atrial natriuretic factor and therapeutic implications. Can J Physiol Pharmacol 69:1576, 1990
21. Dzau VJ, Packer M, Lilly LS et al: Prostaglandins in severe CHF. N Engl J Med 310:347, 1984.
22. Smith TW: Digitalis: mechanisms of action and clinical use. N Engl J Med 318:358, 1988
23. The SOLVD Investigators: Effects of enalapril on survival in patients with reduced left ventricular ejection fractions and congestive heart failure. N Engl J Med 325:293, 1991
24. The CONSENSUS Trial Study Group: Effects of enalapril on mortality in severe congestive heart failure: results of the Cooperative North Scandinavian Enalapril Survival Study (CONSENSUS). N Engl J Med 319:1429, 1987
25. The SOLVD Investigators: Effect of enalapril on mortality and the development of heart failure in asymptomatic patients with reduced left ventricular ejection fractions. N Engl J Med 327:685, 1992
26. Dzau VJ, Hollenberg NK. Renal response to captopril in severe heart failure: role of furosemide in natriuresis and reversal of hyponatremia. Ann Intern Med 100:777, 1984
27. Olsen NV, Hansen JM, Ladefoged SD et al: Renal tubular reabsorption of sodium and water during infusion of low-dose dopamine in normal man. Clin Sci 78:503, 1990
28. Aperia A, Bertorello A, Seri I: Dopamine causes inhibition of Na^+,K^+-ATPase activity in rat proximal convoluted tubule segments. Am J Physiol 252:F39, 1987
29. Bichet DG, Groves BM, Schrier RW: Mechanisms of improvement of water and sodium excretion by immersion in decompensated cirrhotic patients. Kidney Int 24:788, 1983
30. Rosoff L, Zia P, Reynolds T, Horton R: Studies of renin and aldosterone in cirrhotic patients with ascites. Gastroenterology 69:698, 1975
31. Bichet DG, Van Putten VJ, Schrier RW: Potential role of increased sympathetic activity in impaired sodium and water excretion in cirrhosis. N Engl J Med 307:1552, 1982
32. Lieberman FL, Reynolds TB: Plasma volume in cirrhosis of the liver: its relation to portal hypertension, ascites, and renal failure. J Clin Invest 46:1297, 1967
33. Lieberman FL, Ito S, Reynolds TB: Effective plasma volume in cirrhosis with ascites. Evidence that a decreased value does not account for renal sodium retention, a spontaneous reduction in glomerular filtration rate (GFR), and a fall in GFR during drug-induced diuresis. J Clin Invest 48:975, 1969
34. Levy M: Sodium retention and ascites formation in dogs with portal cirrhosis. Am J Physiol 233:F572, 1977

35. Levy M, Wexler MJ: Renal sodium retention and ascites formation in dogs with experimental cirrhosis but without portal hypertension or increased splanchnic vascular capacity. J Lab Clin Med 91:520, 1978

36. Unikowsky B, Wexler MJ, Levy M: Dogs with experimental cirrhosis of the liver but without intrahepatic hypertension do not retain sodium or form ascites. J Clin Invest 72:1594, 1983

37. Schrier RW, Arroyo V, Bernard M et al: Peripheral arterial vasodilation hypothesis: a proposal for the initiation of renal sodium and water retention in cirrhosis. Hepatology 8:1151, 1988

38. Shear L, Ching S, Gabuzda GJ: Compartmentalization of ascites and edema in patients with hepatic cirrhosis. N Engl J Med 282:1391, 1970

39. Perez-Ayuso RM, Arroyo V, Planas R et al: Randomized comparative study of efficacy of furosemide versus spironolactone in nonazotemic cirrhosis with ascites. Gastroenterology 84:961, 1983

40. Pinzani M, Daskalopoulos G, Laffi G et al: Altered furosemide pharmacokinetics in chronic alcoholic liver disease with ascites contributes to diuretic resistance. Gastroenterology 92:294, 1987

41. Inoue M, Okajima K, Itoh K et al: Mechanism of furosemide resistance in analbuminemic rats and hypoalbuminemic patients. Kidney Int 32:198, 1987

42. Pinto PC, Amerian J, Reynolds TB: Large-volume paracentesis in nonedematous patients with tense ascites: its effect on intravascular volume. Hepatology 8:207, 1988

43. Tulassay T, Rascher W, Lang RE et al: Atrial natriuretic peptide and other vasoactive hormones in nephrotic syndrome. Kidney Int 31:1391, 1987

44. Meltzer JI, Keim GH, Laragh JH et al: Nephrotic syndrome: vasoconstriction and hypervolemic types indicated by renin-sodium profiling. Ann Intern Med 91:688, 1979

45. Eisenberg S: Blood volume in persons with the nephrotic syndrome. Am J Med Sci 255:320, 1968

46. Joles JA, Koomans HA, Kortlandt W et al: Hypoproteinemia and recovery from edema in dogs. Am J Physiol 254:F887, 1988

47. Ichikawa I, Bennke HG, Hoyer JR et al: Role for intrarenal mechanisms in the impaired salt excretion of experimental nephrotic syndrome. J Clin Invest 71:91, 1988

48. Guyton AC: Interstitial fluid pressure: II pressure-volume curves of interstitial space. Circ Res 16:452, 1965

49. Taylor EA: Capillary fluid filtration, Starling forces and lymph flow. Circ Res 49:557, 1981

50. Fadnes HO, Reed RK, Aukland K: Mechanisms regulating interstitial fluid volume. Lymphology 11:165, 1978

51. Kirchner KA, Voelker JR, Brater DC: Tubular resistance to furosemide contributes to the attenuated diuretic response in nephrotic rats. J Am Soc Neph 2:1201, 1992

52. Oster JR, Epstein M, Smoller S: Combination therapy with thiazide-type and loop diuretic agents for resistant sodium retention. Ann Intern Med 99:405, 1983

2

Clinical Hyponatremia

Theodore M. Danoff
Eric G. Neilson

Hyponatremia is one of the most common electrolyte disturbances found in clinical medicine. The name, though, is somewhat misleading, because hyponatremia is usually a problem of too much H_2O, not too little sodium. This H_2O excess elicits the physiologically significant consequence of hyponatremia: low osmolality. Osmolality is a measurement of the total number of particles per unit mass of H_2O. The particles are ions like sodium or potassium, or molecules like sugars, lipids, or proteins. When H_2O collects in the body, it dilutes the concentration of these particles, and lowers the osmolality.

Sodium concentration is used as a rough guide to osmolality because it is routinely measured, and because Na is the major contributor to extracellular osmolality. Low serum Na concentration does not reflect total body Na content; rather, it is primarily a measure of body H_2O content relative to solute content (in this case principally Na^+ and K^+ salts), that is, osmolality.

Derangements in osmolality are significant because osmolality regulates cell volume by controlling H_2O movement across the cell membrane. The intracellular space is surrounded by the cell membrane, which separates it from the extracellular compartment. The net movement of H_2O across this membrane is determined by the relative osmolality on each side of the membrane. Water moves from areas of low osmolality (high H_2O concentration) to areas of high osmolality (low H_2O concentration). When extracellular osmolality is low, H_2O moves from the extracellular space into the cells. This added intracellular H_2O causes cell swelling. Osmolality needs to be carefully regulated because normal cell volume is important for proper physiologic function. Osmolality is regulated by controlling the amount of H_2O in the body. Accordingly, the understanding and treatment of hyponatremia requires an understanding of H_2O metabolism.

PHYSIOLOGY OF H_2O METABOLISM

Changes in total body H_2O represent the difference between H_2O intake and H_2O excretion. The principal source of H_2O intake is oral fluids, while the principal source of H_2O excretion is urine. In hospitalized patients, intravenous fluids are often a major source of H_2O intake that is not under physiologic control.

25

The physiologic stimulus for H_2O intake is thirst. Thirst stimuli are primarily increases in serum osmolality and decreases in effective arterial blood volume. The increased serum osmolality is detected by osmoreceptors in the hypothalamus. The decreased effective arterial blood volume (EABV) is detected by baroreceptors located in the left atrium and carotid bodies, and by the juxtaglomerular apparatus (JGA). The baroreceptors signal via neurons, whereas the JGA signals use the renin-angiotensin pathway. Decreased effective arterial blood volume stimulates renin release by the JGA. The renin stimulates the conversion of angiotensinogen to angiotensin I, which is subsequently converted to angiotensin II (AII). Angiotensin II is a potent thirst stimulant (dipsogen).

The kidneys normally rid the body of any excess H_2O, aside from a relatively small amount of insensible H_2O loss (about 7 mL/kg/day). Hyponatremia develops when H_2O intake exceeds H_2O excretion. The steps involved in renal excretion of H_2O are the formation of a filtrate, the extraction of salt from the filtrate to form a dilute urine, and the excretion of this dilute urine. Under appropriate conditions, the renal capacity to excrete H_2O is substantial (about 20 L/day). Factors that interfere with any of these steps can substantially reduce the kidneys' ability to excrete H_2O. Figure 2-1 shows a stylized nephron and indicates the location and extent of dilute urine formation.

The initial volume of filtrate depends on the glomerular filtration rate (GFR). The filtrate is then delivered to the proximal convoluted tubule where 65% to 90% of it is reabsorbed in an isotonic fashion. The amount reabsorbed depends primarily on the EABV. Conditions of decreased EABV favor increased proximal tubular reabsorption of Na and H_2O. Increased proximal reabsorption results in decreased delivery of H_2O to the distal nephron. This inevitably results in a reduction in the amount of H_2O that the kidneys can excrete. The variation in proximal reabsorption based on effective arterial blood volume is one of the major determinants of H_2O excretion.

The thin, descending limb of Henle is slightly H_2O permeable, so H_2O gets extracted from the filtrate as the thin limb passes through the hypertonic medulla. The thick, ascending limb is H_2O impermeable, so no H_2O is removed, although NaCl is extracted. This results in the formation of a dilute urine. Further urinary dilution occurs in the distal convoluted tubule.

Dilute urine enters the collecting tubules that pass through the hypertonic medulla. The H_2O permeability of the collecting tubules is regulated by antidiuretic hormone (ADH). When ADH is present, the tubules become H_2O permeable and H_2O is drawn out of the lumen of the collecting tubule and into the medulla. As can be seen from Figure 2-1, when ADH is present, 10 to 20 liters of free H_2O can be reabsorbed in the collecting tubules, essentially resulting in no urinary free-H_2O clearance.

In Figure 2-1, the tonicity of the filtrate as it moves along the nephron is indicated. The changes in tonicity reflect extraction of salt and/or water from the filtrate. To help conceptualize the factors that effect urinary free-H_2O clearance, the table below the schematic gives an idealized set of urine volumes that pass through the nephron under different states of volume repletion and renal function. Free-H_2O clearance can never be greater than the volume of urine; therefore, factors that stimulate reabsorption of the filtrate decrease free-H_2O clearance. The formation of the filtrate at the glomeruli is the first step in the excretion of free H_2O. As can be seen in the column listing the volume of filtrate formation, significant filtrate volumes are formed even with a markedly reduced GFR. The amount of urine reabsorbed in the proximal tubule is one of the major determinants of urinary free-H_2O clearance. The EABV also influences the volume reabsorbed in this segment. As EABV decreases, the percent reabsorbed increases from about 65% to 90% of the volume entering the descending limb. The urine becomes hypertonic as it

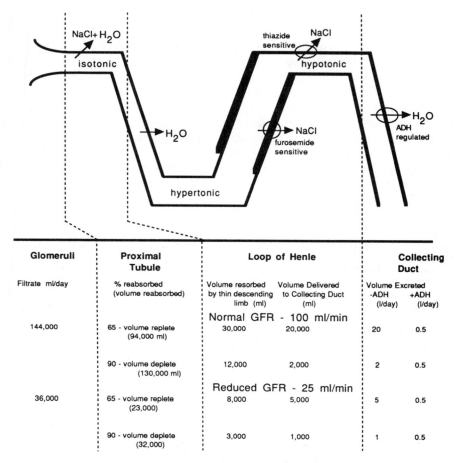

Glomeruli	Proximal Tubule	Loop of Henle		Collecting Duct	
Filtrate ml/day	% reabsorbed (volume reabsorbed)	Volume resorbed by thin descending limb (ml)	Volume Delivered to Collecting Duct (ml)	Volume Excreted -ADH (l/day)	+ADH (l/day)
		Normal GFR - 100 ml/min			
144,000	65 - volume replete (94,000 ml)	30,000	20,000	20	0.5
	90 - volume deplete (130,000 ml)	12,000	2,000	2	0.5
		Reduced GFR - 25 ml/min			
36,000	65 - volume replete (23,000)	8,000	5,000	5	0.5
	90 - volume deplete (32,000)	3,000	1,000	1	0.5

Fig. 2-1. A schematic diagram of the nephron with the segments of the nephron critical to water metabolism marked (see text for details).

travels through the thin descending limb because of the H_2O extraction. As it travels through the H_2O impermeable thick ascending limb and NaCl is reabsorbed, the urine becomes progressively more hypotonic. The actual rate of free H_2O clearance depends on the volume of hypotonic urine that reaches the collecting duct. The collecting duct is water impermeable in the absence of ADH, but becomes very permeable in response to ADH stimulation. With no ADH present ($-$ADH), free-H_2O clearance approaches the volume delivered to the collecting duct. In the presence of ADH ($+$ADH), the urine output drops to approximately 500 mL. This is the minimal volume required to clear the bodies obligate solute load. This 500 mL represents almost no free-H_2O clearance.

The major determinants for urinary free-H_2O excretion are (1) *Effective arterial blood volume,* which effects proximal urinary reabsorption, hence distal urinary delivery; and (2) *ADH status,* which effects the reabsorption of the dilute urine in the collecting ducts. Mindful consideration of these two factors is critical in evaluating every case of hyponatremia.

OSMOLALITY AND TONICITY

The osmotic pressure that determines H_2O movement is defined as the number of particles (e.g., amino acids, sugars, and ions) relative to the number of H_2O molecules. Water moves across the cell membrane to balance osmotic pressures. Some particles remain primarily extracellular and determine extracellular osmotic pressure (Na, glucose, albumin). Some particles are primarily intracellular (K and proteins of the cell). Some particles, like urea, can easily move across the cell membrane so their extracellular concentration equals their intracellular concentration, and they exert no transmembrane osmotic pressure gradient. The term *tonicity* refers to the osmotic pressure of solutes that stay only on one side of the membrane, and therefore cause H_2O movement by exerting a transmembrane osmotic pressure gradient. Those osmoles that cause changes in tonicity are called *effective osmoles;* those that easily cross the membrane are called *ineffective osmoles.*

Effective Osmoles (Solutes)	*Ineffective Osmoles (Solutes)*
NaCl (extracellular)	Urea
Glucose, mannitol (extracellular)	Ethanol
KCl (intracellular)	

Only effective osmoles contribute to tonicity, whereas all solutes contribute to osmolality. Tonicity and osmolality can be calculated by

$$\text{Tonicity} = Na^+(mEq/L) \times 2 + \frac{mg/dL \text{ glucose}}{18} + \frac{\text{Any effective osmole (mg/dL)}}{\text{mol wt of the effective osmole}/10} \qquad \text{(Eq. 2-1)}$$

$$\text{Osmolality} = Na^+(mEq/L) \times 2 + \frac{mg/dL \text{ glucose}}{18} + \frac{mg/dL \text{ BUN}}{2.8} + \frac{\text{Every solute (mg/dL)}}{\text{mol wt of the solute}/10} \qquad \text{(Eq. 2-2)}$$

TONICITY AND HYPONATREMIA

Although Na is the primary extracellular solute, there are other solutes that contribute to tonicity. Therefore, hyponatremia can occur in the setting of high, normal, or low tonicity. The first step in evaluating any case of hyponatremia is to estimate the tonicity of the patient's plasma.

Isotonic Hyponatremia

Isotonic hyponatremia, also called pseudohyponatremia, is a laboratory artifact that occurs in the setting of extreme hyperlipidemia or hyperproteinemia. Plasma normally is about 93% aqueous and 7% proteins and lipids. If the clinical laboratory uses instrumentation that reports Na content per unit volume plasma rather than Na content per volume of the aqueous phase, then

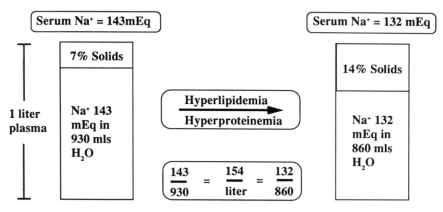

Fig. 2-2. A schematic depiction of why hyperlipidemia or hyperproteinemia causes falsely low measured serum Na by some analytic techniques (see text for details). (Modified from Narins RG, Jones ER, Stom MC, Rudnick MR, Bastl CP: Diagnostic strategies in disorders of fluid, electrolyte and acid-base homeostasis. Am J Med 72:496, 1982

significant elevations in lipid or protein content can cause the reported Na value to be artificially low. This is schematically depicted in Figure 2-2.

Basically, two types of instruments are used in clinical laboratories to determine serum Na concentrations: ion-specific electrodes and flame photometers. Ion-specific electrodes measure the Na concentration in the aqueous phase. The normal Na concentration in the aqueous phase of plasma is 154 mEq/L. The nonaqueous phase of plasma is Na free and occupies approximately 7% of the plasma volume, hence the normal Na concentration in the aqueous phase is 143 mEq/ L (93% aqueous × 154 + 7% nonaqueous × 0 = 143). Laboratories that utilize ion-specific electrodes for Na measurement assume that the nonaqueous phase is always 7%, therefore this laboratory value is unaffected by increases in the nonaqueous phase. The lipids and proteins in the nonaqueous phase are high molecular weight molecules, hence the nonaqueous phase does not contribute significantly to the plasma osmolality.

Flame photometers on the other hand measure Na content per volume of plasma. When the nonaqueous phase increases, then the flame photometer reports a decreased Na concentration. As indicated in Figure 2-2, if the nonaqueous phase increases to 14% of the plasma volume, then the flame photometer reports a Na concentration of 132 mEq/L (86% aqueous × 154 + 14% nonaqueous × 0 = 132). Although the plasma tonicity has not changed, the flame photometer is reporting a low serum Na concentration despite normal Na concentration in the aqueous phase.

This laboratory artifact will be significant only in the presence of severe hyperlipidemia (plasma will look milky) or hyperproteinemia (>15 mg/dL). Laboratories using flame photometers (or diluting electrodes) are affected by this problem, whereas direct ion-specific electrodes are not. Fortunately, these clinical conditions are rare and most clinical laboratories do not use the former types of machines. A direct measurement of osmolality (by freezing point depression) will confirm a normal serum osmolality in spite of a low osmolality calculated from the serum Na concentration. The Na concentration in the aqueous phase is not changed by the addition of the lipids or proteins; therefore, the tonicity is normal and cell volume is not affected. This condition does not cause clinical symptoms of hypotonicity.

Hypertonic Hyponatremia

Hypertonic hyponatremia, also called factitious hyponatremia, occurs when effective solutes are added to the extracellular fluid. Plasma osmolality in these cases is high. The low serum Na concentration is caused by the redistribution of H_2O from the intracellular compartent to the extracellular compartment, which equalizes the tonicity. Total body H_2O remains constant, but is redistributed from the intracellular space to the extracellular space. This clinical condition can be seen with hyperglycemia in diabetes mellitus, and in patients given mannitol to lower intracranial pressure. A direct measurement of osmolality will confirm an elevated serum osmolality in spite of the low serum Na value. The clinical symptoms produced by this condition are related to the hypertonicity, not the hyponatremia.

Hypotonic Hyponatremia

Hypotonic hyponatremia is the clinically significant case when plasma tonicity is low (<280 mOsm/L). The hyponatremia is due to an excess of H_2O relative to the absolute content of Na. The low tonicity reflects too much H_2O, not too little Na. The clinical symptoms are always due to the ingestion or administration of H_2O coupled with a failure to excrete that H_2O.

FREE H_2O EXCRETION

The kidneys are the body's primary means of H_2O excretion. Hypotonic hyponatremia occurs when the kidneys cannot excrete a sufficient quantity of H_2O. The urine contains a wide range of solutes and electrolytes. For this reason, urine output does not equal H_2O output. The urinary H_2O output is termed free-H_2O clearance, and is best calculated by only considering effective osmols as solutes. The most abundant effective osmols in urine are Na^+ and K^+. In patients with hyponatremia, the volume of electrolyte-free H_2O is the only important volume in determining water balance. Mathematically,

Total urine output = Volume of electrolyte-free urine

+ Volume of urine with an electrolyte content equal to that of the serum   (Eq. 2-3)

The free-H_2O clearance is calculated as follows:

Free-H_2O clearance = Urine volume × $(1 - \text{urine } (Na^+ + K^+)/\text{serum } (Na^+ + K^+))$ (Eq. 2-4)

For example, if the serum $[Na^+] = 145$ mEq/L and $[K^+] = 5.0$ mEq/L and the 24-hour urine has a volume of 2 liters and an electrolyte concentration of $[Na^+] = 45$ mEq/L and $[K^+] = 30$ mEq/L, then the kidneys can be thought to excrete 1.5 liters of electrolyte-free urine and 0.5 liter of urine with an electrolyte concentration of 150 mmol/L. In this case the free-H_2O clearance is 1.5 liters.

Free H_2O can also take on a negative value when urine (Na + K) is greater than serum (Na + K). The consequence of a negative free-H_2O clearance is that the more urine the patient excretes, the more hyponatremic the patient will become. For example, if the patient weighed 70 kg and had a serum $[Na^+]$ of 145 mEq/L and $[K^+]$ of 5.0 mEq/L, a 24-hour urine volume of 2 liters and an electrolyte concentration of $[Na^+]$ of 150 mEq/L and $[K^+]$ of 50 mEq/L, then the free-H_2O clearance is

$$\text{Free-}H_2O \text{ clearance} = 2 \text{ L} \times (1 - (150 + 50)/(145 + 5)) \qquad \text{(Eq. 2-5)}$$
$$= -0.67 \text{ L}$$

The kidneys can be thought to have generated 0.67 liters of water. The result of a negative free-H_2O clearance is that the hyponatremia worsens as more urine is made.

CLINICAL SETTINGS OF HYPOTONIC HYPONATREMIA

Clinically, cases of hyponatremia can be divided into three categories based on total body Na. Total body Na reflects the patient's volume status, although not necessarily EABV. There are three clinical categories, and an overview of the classification is shown in Figure 2-3.

Sodium Deficient/Volume Depletion

The clinical findings in this category are tachycardia, weight loss, and changes in orthostatic vital signs. Volume depletion leads to a decreased EABV and increased proximal tubular reabsorption of Na and H_2O, which results in inadequate urine delivery to the diluting segment. Second, volume depletion is a stimuli for ADH release, causing reabsorption of free H_2O in the collecting tubules. Finally, volume depletion stimulates thirst, which promotes H_2O ingestion.

Sodium Excess/Volume Overload

Here the clinical findings are peripheral edema and pulmonary edema (heart failure). The pathophysiology is generally due to decreased EABV in spite of total body volume overload. The decreased EABV (decreased renal perfusion) produces the same effect as volume depletion

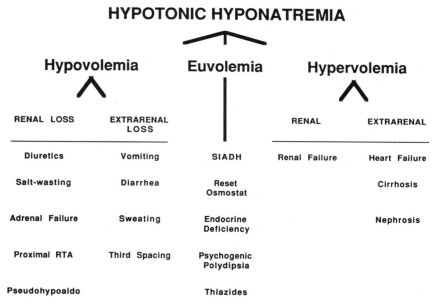

Fig. 2-3. Differential diagnosis for hypotonic hyponatremia. The patients are categorized based on their volume status. This division uses the clinical exam findings of orthostasis, edema, and signs of heart failure to divide the patient population. Under the hypovolemic heading, the patients are divided by the route of the Na loss. Under the hypervolemic heading, the patients are divided by the etiology of their Na retentive state.

with increased proximal Na and H_2O reabsorption, as well as elevated ADH levels. In the case of renal failure, the decreased GFR limits the renal clearance of free H_2O.

Euvolemic

The clinical findings are no edema and no orthostatic vital sign changes. Pathophysiology is generally due to levels of ADH inappropriate for a given serum osmolality.

CLINICAL MANIFESTATIONS OF HYPOTONIC HYPONATREMIA

The clinical findings in hypotonic hyponatremia depend on the magnitude of the hypotonicity as well as the rapidity of its development. A symptom complex including headache, apathy, nausea, vomiting, abdominal cramps, confusion, muscle twitching, seizures, and coma can be seen. Acute H_2O intoxication of less than 24 hours often presents with symptoms at Na levels beginning at 125 mEq/L. Seizures and coma appear in acute hyponatremia with Na levels below 115 mEq/L. Chronic hyponatremia is often asymptomatic until the Na concentration drops below 115 mEq/L.

The brain is the organ most noticeably affected by changes in tonicity. If H_2O movement to equalize transmembrane osmotic pressures were the brain's sole mode of osmotic compensation, small changes in tonicity, regardless of the rapidity, would have significant consequences. The brain, however, has several mechanisms that help it adapt to decreased extracellular osmolality, other than swelling up and herniating through the foramen magnum. Cell swelling causes an increase in interstitial pressure, which increases the flow of fluid into the CSF. The brain cells also have intrinsic defense mechanisms. They lose intracellular potassium and "idiogenic osmoles," which lowers the intracellular osmolality. Idiogenic osmoles are no longer idiopathic and are now recognized to be amino acids, polyols, and methylamines. Potassium efflux from brain cells is first measured 3 to 4 hours after the osmotic change, and is maximal in less than 24 hours. The loss of idiogenic osmoles occurs over several days. Through increased CSF production and decreased intracellular osmolality, brain cell swelling in hypotonic states is minimized, assuming the change is slow enough to allow compensation.

In the chronic hypotonic state, brain cells adapt to the decreased tonicity, and the patient is often asymptomatic. It is important to correct the hypotonicity slowly, because the adaptive process leaves the brain cells susceptible to shrinkage as the external milieu becomes hypertonic in comparison. Correction that is too rapid and overcorrection have been associated with an osmotic demyelinating syndrome (central pontine myelinolysis). These patients undergo gradual neurologic deterioration one to several days after the correction of the hypotonic state. Central pontine myelinolysis can present as pseudobulbar palsy and quadriparesis with swallowing dysfunction and inability to speak. Sometimes these symptoms improve, but some patients are left with significant permanent sequelae.

MANAGEMENT OF HYPOTONIC HYPONATREMIA

The management of patients with hypotonic hyponatremia requires two considerations: (1) correction of the pathophysiology leading to the hypotonic state, and (2) correction of the hypotonic state.

As discussed above, the abnormality in the hypotonic state is an imbalance of H_2O intake and output. To correct the problem, both sides of the balance can be addressed. Water intake can be restricted. If H_2O intake is totally stopped, hypotonicity cannot get worse. To correct the output problem, the factors reducing urinary free-H_2O excretion must be corrected. The factors that are generally amenable to clinical manipulation are (1) repleting the intravascular volume if the patient is hypovolemic, (2) stopping medications that augment ADH action or release, (3) correcting hypothyroidism or hypoadrenalism, and (4) improving cardiac output if the patient has heart failure. Obviously, the clinical setting of the hypotonic state will guide the management approach.

The correction of the hypotonic state must be guided by the patient's symptoms. If the patient is asymptomatic, correction of the pathology causing the hypotonic state and watchful waiting may very well be enough. If the patient is symptomatic, more active intervention is needed.

If symptomatic hypotonic hyponatremia develops acutely (<12 h), then hypertonic saline (usually 3%), infused at a rate designed to increase the serum Na level by 1 mEq/L/h, is used. This infusion should continue until the patient becomes asymptomatic or a serum Na level of 120 mEq/L is attained, at which point the hypertonic saline infusion is discontinued. The serum Na should not be elevated by more than 25 mEq/L during the first 48 hours of therapy. Because the brain has not had time to adapt to the hypotonic state, rapid correction will not result in significant cell shrinkage and therefore is relatively safe, assuming the patient's cardiovascular system can tolerate the addition of salts to the extravascular space. The calculation of hypertonic replacement is as follows:

$$\text{Total Body } H_2O = 60\% \times \text{Body weight in kg} \qquad \text{(Eq. 2-6)}$$

$$\text{Salt replacement} = (120 - \text{Actual serum Na}^+) \times \text{body } H_2O \qquad \text{(Eq. 2-7)}$$

$$\text{Volume of hypertonic saline} = \frac{\text{Salt replacement}}{\text{Na}^+ \text{ content of 3\% saline}} \qquad \text{(Eq. 2-8)}$$

Substituting

$$\text{Volume of hypertonic saline} = \frac{(120 - \text{Actual serum Na}^+) \times 0.60 \times \text{Wt in kg}}{513 \text{ mEq/L}} \qquad \text{(Eq. 2-9)}$$

Trouble develops when hypotonic hyponatremia is discovered and is thought to be acute but is actually chronic (>12 h duration). In chronic hyponatremia the cells of the brain have had time to adapt to the hypotonic state, so rapid correction can result in cell shrinkage and possibly an osmotic demyelinating disorder. If in doubt about the duration of the hypotonic state, treat the patient as if the hyponatremia were chronic.

The level of aggressiveness of treatment of chronic hypotonic hyponatremia will depend on the severity of the symptoms.

For severe symptoms such as coma, seizures, and significant change in mental status (confusion) the treatment should include

1. Hypertonic saline over 2 to 3 hours to increase $[\text{Na}^+]$ by up to 5 mEq/L or until symptoms resolve. The volume of hypertonic saline can be calculated as in Equation 2-9. Furosemide may be needed to prevent pulmonary edema or heart failure, but care must be taken to also avoid volume depletion secondary to overaggressive diuresis.
2. After the hypertonic infusion, the intravenous fluid is changed to 0.9% saline and furosemide is given to keep urine output equal to intravenous fluid infusion rate. The furosemide is given to inhibit the kidneys' ability to generate a concentrated urine, because under certain conditions (e.g., high ADH) urine (Na + K) can exceed 154 mEq/L (Na concentration in 0.9% saline). In these cases, the patient can have a net H_2O gain (become more hyponatremic)

despite receiving only saline, because the urinary free-H_2O clearance is negative. For this reason, it is worth checking urine electrolytes during therapy to assure that the patient has a positive urinary free-H_2O clearance. Follow serum Na frequently and adjust infusion rate as needed. Remember that the patient has ongoing H_2O loss (insensible plus urinary free-H_2O clearance), which can cause serum Na to rise faster than expected or desired.

3. Generally, correct serum Na no faster than 0.5 to 1.0 mEq/L/h to a Na of 125 to 130 mEq/ L.

Moderate symptoms include mild changes in mental status (headache). A 0.9% saline solution with furosemide diuresis is often a convenient approach. Correct Na no faster than 0.5 to 1.0 mEq/L/h and aim to correct the Na no higher than 125 to 130 mEq/L.

If the patient has mild or no symptoms, H_2O restriction is enough.

One of the major difficulties in managing hyponatremia is controlling the rate of rise of the serum Na. Although body H_2O and Na deficit calculations are accurate, there are ongoing H_2O losses from the urine and insensible evaporation. These are hard to account for. Frequent follow-up of the patient's status and repeat serum Na measurements are necessary. A spot measurement of urine electrolytes can help in estimating urinary free-H_2O clearance.

GENERAL READINGS

Anderson RJ, Chung HM, Rudiger K, Schrier RW: Hyponatremia: a prospective analysis of its epidemiology and the pathogenetic role of vasopressin. Ann Intern Med 102:164, 1985

Berl T: Treating hyponatremia: damned if we do and damned if we don't. Kidney Int 37:1006, 1990

Cooke CR, Turin MD, Walker WG: The syndrome of inappropriate antidiuretic hormone secretion (SIADH): pathophysiologic mechanisms in solute and volume regulation. Medicine 58:240, 1979

Moses AM, Miller M: Drug-induced dilutional hyponatremia. N Engl J Med 291:1234, 1974

Rose BD: New approach to disturbances in the plasma sodium concentration. Am J Med 81:1033, 1986

CASE STUDY 1

Hyponatremia Associated with Volume Depletion

A 23-year-old medical student, Joe Tilt, developed profuse watery diarrhea while doing a third year clinical clerkship. He drank a variety of juices to speed his recovery, but, despite good oral intake, he eventually became lightheaded upon standing. He presented to his intern, who evaluated him. He reported that his usual weight is 75 kg.

During his physical examination, his blood pressure was 84/64 mmHg and pulse 120 while standing; while lying down, blood pressure was 100/60 and pulse was 100. His temperature was 38°C, present weight was 70 kg, and chest and heart normal. His abdomen was soft with active bowel sounds. The stool was heme negative.

LABORATORY DATA

Na 129 mEq/L	CO_2 20 mEq/L	Creatinine 1.0 mg/dL
K 3.0 mEq/L	BUN 20 mg/dL	Glucose 94 mg/dL
Cl 92 mEq/L		

Urine chemistries: Na 5 mEq/L, Cl 10 mEq/L, and osm 520 mOsm/kg.

Question 1. Compared to his normal state, what is his relative body sodium content?

Question 2. What is the calculated serum osmolality?

Question 3. Explain the pathophysiology causing the hyponatremia in this patient.

Question 4. How would you treat this patient?

---

1. Compared to his normal state, what is his relative body sodium content?

The patient is volume depleted and therefore must be Na depleted. Evidence for the volume depletion includes reduced body weight and orthostatic changes in heart rate and blood pressure. The low urinary Na is consistent with the kidneys being in a Na-avid state because of a decreased EABV. Orthostatic changes in heart rate and blood pressure are consistent with at least 10% volume depletion. Mr. Tilt's 5-kg loss of body weight is consistent with the 10% volume depletion and indicates he needs approximately 5 L of 0.9% saline to correct the volume depletion. The hyponatremia is not an indicator of body sodium content.

2. What is the calculated serum osmolality?

$$\text{Serum osm} = 2 \times \text{Na}^+ + \frac{\text{BUN}}{2.8} + \frac{\text{Glu}}{18}$$

$$= 2 \times 129 + \frac{20}{2.8} + \frac{94}{18} \qquad \text{(Eq. 2-10)}$$

$$= 270 \text{ mOsm/kg}$$

However, since urea is not an effective osmolyte, the tonicity is only 263.

3. Explain the pathophysiology causing the hyponatremia in this patient.

This patient has both volume depletion and H_2O excess. This situation developed from Na loss through diarrhea, with repletion using low Na solutions. Normally the H_2O excess would be cleared by the kidney, but the regulation of H_2O metabolism has been disrupted by the volume depletion. Volume depletion (decreased EABV) stimulates proximal tubular salt and H_2O reabsorption; therefore, less fluid is delivered distally to the thick ascending limb and distal tubule where urine dilution occurs. With less volume of distal urine delivery, less dilute urine can be made. Dilution of tubular fluid is the way the kidney disposes of excess free H_2O. The volume depletion is also a stimulus for ADH release. In the presence of ADH, free H_2O generated in the distal tubule is reabsorbed in the collecting tubule. This inability to excrete free H_2O coupled with H_2O ingestion causes hyponatremia.

Patients with GI distress also have nausea, which is a potent stimulus of ADH release and can also contribute to the hyponatremia. Mr. Tilt denied nausea. Hypotonicity will not develop unless the patient drinks or is administered free H_2O under conditions in which the kidneys cannot excrete free H_2O normally.

4. How would you treat this patient?

The reason for reduced free-H_2O clearance is volume depletion; therefore, once this is corrected the kidneys should excrete the excess free H_2O. Based on the physical examination, we estimated the patient to be at least 10% volume depleted. For Mr. Tilt, that would represent 70 kg × 60% (percentage of body weight that is water) × 10% deplete = 4.2 L of 0.9% saline. This approximates his 5 kg weight loss.

CASE STUDY 2

Hyponatremia Associated with Hyperglycemia

Mr. John Sweet, a 72-year-old man with recent onset non-insulin dependent diabetes, presented to the clinic for routine follow-up. His only medication was chlorpropamide 250 mg p.o. b.i.d., which was started 2 weeks earlier. He was without complaint.

Upon physical examination, his temperature was 98.6°, blood pressure was 130/70, and heart rate was 72 without orthostatic changes; weight 165 lbs (baseline weight 165). Lungs and heart were normal. The extremities were without edema, and the neurologic exam was normal.

LABORATORY DATA

Na 127 mEq/L	Glucose 400 mg/dL
K 4.2 mEq/L	Plasma osm 280 mOsm/kg
Cl 89 mEq/L	Urine osm 525 mOsm/kg
CO_2 24 mEq/L	Uric Acid 1.5 mg/dL
BUN 5 mg/dL	Cholesterol 220 mg/dL
Creatinine 0.8 mg/dL	TG 165 mg/dL

Question 1. How does hyperglycemia influence the interpretation of hyponatremia?
Question 2. Calculate the patient's free-H_2O excess.
Question 3. Why is Mr. Sweet hyponatremic?
Question 4. What is the significance of the low uric acid?
Question 5. How should this case be managed?
Question 6. After appropriate therapeutic interventions are implemented, he returns for a follow-up visit. His exam remains unchanged but now his laboratory studies show Na 133 mEq/L, glucose 125 mg/dL, and creatinine 0.8 mg/dL, with a plasma osm of 290 mOsm/kg and a urine osm of 525 mOsm/kg. A review of the old clinic records indicate Mr. Sweet's sodium has been between 133–136 mEq/L and plasma osm 285–295 mOsm/kg since he was first seen in the clinic 3 years earlier. What are the possible etiologies of this persistent hyponatremia?

---

1. How does hyperglycemia influence the interpretation of hyponatremia?

His hyponatremia needs to be interpreted in the context of serum tonicity. When effective solutes are added to the serum they raise tonicity. This rise in tonicity draws H_2O out of cells, leading to a dilution of the Na in the plasma. In this case, the glucose is a tonically effective osmol. A rough rule of thumb is that for every 100 mg/dL of glucose greater than 200 mg/dL the serum Na is depressed by 1.8 mEq/L. In this case the "corrected" Na is closer to 131 mEq/L.

$$\text{corrected Na}^+: 127 + (400 - 200)/100 \times 1.8 = 131 \text{ mEq/L} \qquad \text{(Eq. 2-11)}$$

When Na is corrected for elevated glucose, the patient is still hyponatremic, which, of course, is expected given the lowish plasma osmolality.

At the bedside, one is often faced with low Na sodium values without measured plasma osmolalities. It is critical to calculate the serum tonicity to confirm you are dealing with hypotonic hyponatremia.

If in this case the glucose had been 1,500 mg/dL, the serum osmolality would have been approximately 337 mOsm/kg. That value would suggest that you are dealing with *hypertonic* hyponatremia, which has a very different etiology and management.

2. Calculate the patient's free-H_2O excess.

Free-H_2O excess represents the volume of H_2O that has diluted the patient's Na. When the Na content of the body is held constant, it can be calculated as follows

$$H_2O \text{ excess} = \text{Present body } H_2O - \text{appropriate body } H_2O \qquad \text{(Eq. 2-12)}$$

$$\text{Appropriate body } H_2O \times \text{normal serum Na}^+ = \text{Present body } H_2O \times \text{present serum Na}^+ \qquad \text{(Eq. 2-13)}$$

Rearranging and substituting

$$H_2O \text{ excess} = \text{Present body } H_2O - \frac{\text{Present Body } H_2O \times \text{Present serum Na}^+}{\text{Normal Serum Na}^+} \qquad \text{(Eq. 2-14)}$$

$$H_2O \text{ excess} = \text{Present body } H_2O \ (1 - \text{present serum Na}^+/\text{normal serum Na}^+) \qquad \text{(Eq. 2-15)}$$

Body H_2O is approximately 60% of body weight, therefore,

$$H_2O \text{ excess} = \text{weight} \times 0.6 \ (1 - \text{present serum Na}^+/140) \qquad \text{(Eq. 2-16)}$$

$$H_2O \text{ excess} = (165 \text{ lb}/2.2 \text{ lb/kg}) \times 0.6 \times [1 - (127/140)] = 4.2 \text{ L} \qquad \text{(Eq. 2-17)}$$

3. Why is Mr. Sweet hyponatremic?

Based on the physical findings of no orthostatic changes, no edema and a baseline weight, this patient falls into the category of euvolemic hypotonic hyponatremia. The differential diagnosis for this abnormality includes psychogenic polydipsia, endocrine abnormalities, thiazide-induced hyponatremia, SIADH, or reset osmostat.

To develop hyponatremia from psychogenic polydipsia requires a H_2O intake of usually greater than 10 to 20 liters a day (i.e., an amount greater than the kidney's capacity to excrete excess water). Such patients have very dilute urine. This patient does not have a very dilute urine, as indicated by the urine osm of 525 mOsm/kg (normal for an individual ingesting excess water would be <66 mOsm/kg). Therefore, this diagnosis is unlikely.

Severe hypothyroidism or cortisol deficiency can cause euvolemic hyponatremia. Hypothyroidism causes hyponatremia by decreasing cardiac output, leading to decreased GFR with decreased distal delivery of Na and H_2O to diluting sites. Also thyroid hormone is probably needed to suppress ADH release in the presence of hypotonia. Cortisol is also needed to suppress ADH in the presence of hypotonia. The patient does not have findings of hypothyroidism (hung reflexes, hypothermia, bradycardia, or the electrolyte abnormalities of hypoadrenalism: hyper K), which makes these diagnoses less likely.

The patient does not take thiazide or thiazide-like diuretics, ruling out the diagnosis of thiazide-induced hyponatremia. Since some patients take diuretics surreptitiously for weight loss or edema control, this should be kept in mind if a history of weight consciousness or unusual body-image consciousness is elicited.

The syndrome of inappropriate antidiuretic hormone secretion (SIADH), as the name implies, results in increased ADH levels in the euvolemic but hypotonic state. It is a diagnosis of exclusion. The diagnosis requires

euvolemia
hypotonicity of body fluids
normal renal function
normal thyroid and adrenal function
normal cardiac function
urine osm > plasma osm or a urine osm inappropriately elevated for the level of plasma osm

The causes of SIADH include

pain and anxiety
CNS disease (tumor, trauma, meningitis)
pulmonary disease (tumor, asthma, pneumonia)
drugs (chlorpropamide, cytoxan, clofibrate, cyclophosphamide, vincristine)
psychotropics (navane, prolixin, mellaril)

This patient's oral hypoglycemic medication, chlorpropamide, causes SIADH by stimulating ADH release. This patient is euvolemic, has normal cardiac, renal, and adrenal function and has a urine osm greater than plasma osm; therefore, SIADH is the most likely diagnosis.

4. What is the significance of the low uric acid?

Patients with SIADH are subclinically volume overloaded because of a slight water excess. Low uric acid is an indicator of the patient's volume status (renal excretion of uric acid rises with ECF expansion); therefore, low uric acids with high fractional excretions of uric acid are consistent with SIADH. The patients low BUN/creatinine ratio is also consistent with a volume replete state.

5. How should this case be managed?

The patient is volume replete and has no symptoms from the hyponatremia. Discontinuing the chlorpropamide with H_2O restriction should be adequate therapy. In this case, an alternate means of controlling the patient's diabetes mellitus, such as a second generation oral hypoglycemic agent, will have to be used. Glucose control will be important, because the osmotic diuresis induced by hyperglycemia can lead to volume depletion, which can interfere with normal H_2O metabolism.

6. What are the possible etiologies of this persistent hyponatremia?

Persistent hyponatremia in spite of discontinuation of the chlorpropamide raises the question of a reset osmostat. Clinically, such patients appear to have SIADH. Their pituitary gland seems to have altered its threshold for ADH release. They excrete a normal H_2O load, but return to a lower serum osmolality. A reset osmostat does not seem to be physiologically significant.

CASE STUDY 3

Hyponatremia Associated with Thiazide Use

Miss Matty Caishun, a 70-year-old woman, was noted to have mild systolic hypertension when she was seen in the clinic. Her laboratory studies were notable for a Na level of 140 mEq/L and a creatinine level of 1.0 mg/dL. Her physical examination revealed a weight of 45 kg, normal heart and lung exam, and no peripheral edema. She was started on hydrochlorothiazide 50 mg/day and amiloride 5 mg/day. She returned to the clinic four days later, complaining of confusion.

Her physical examination at that time reveals blood pressure of 152/84 mmHg (previous blood pressure was 172/90), and pulse of 82 without orthostatic changes. The JVP is approximately 5 cm at 30°. Her chest is clear, cardiac exam unremarkable, and there is no peripheral edema. The neurologic exam shows her to be lethargic and confused.

LABORATORY DATA

Na 120 mEq/L	BUN 25 mg/dL	Plasma osm 245 mOsm/kg
K 4.0 mEq/L	Creatinine 1.1 mg/dL	Urinary osm 590 mOsm/kg
Cl 75 mEq/L	Glucose 135 mg/dL	Urinary Na 35 mEq/L
CO_2 30 mEq/L		

Question 1. What is the most likely etiology of the hyponatremia, and what is its pathophysiology?
Question 2. What is the best therapy?
Question 3. What advice would you give her to avoid this problem in the future?

---

1. What is the most likely etiology of the hyponatremia, and what is its pathophysiology?

Miss Caishun's profound hyponatremia developed soon after the initiation of therapy with a thiazide diuretic. Thiazide-induced hyponatremia is therefore the most likely etiology. Only a very small percentage of patients started on thiazides develop profound hyponatremia, but those that do share certain common characteristics. These characteristics include female gender, age greater than 60 years, small body size, and a large baseline fluid intake. When the thiazides are started, several different steps in H_2O metabolism are disrupted. The thiazides cause a sodium diuresis, which leads to subclinical volume depletion. This volume depletion promotes salt and H_2O reabsorption in the proximal tubule. When proximal reabsorption is increased, there is decreased distal delivery of fluid, so less free H_2O can be cleared. In the distal nephron, the reabsorption of Na in the diluting segments is inhibited by the thiazide, so the urine that escapes the proximal tubule cannot be maximally dilute. Finally, in some patients, ADH is not maximally suppressed, possibly a result of subclinical volume depletion, and urinary free H_2O that reaches the collecting tubules is reabsorbed. There is some evidence that such patients are also potassium depleted intracellularly, and this potassium depletion may promote a higher than normal intracellular Na content.

2. What is the best therapy?

Given that Miss Caishun is moderately symptomatic, a reasonable management strategy would include discontinuation of the thiazide diuretic, oral fluid restriction, and administration of 0.9% saline. If there is concern that the patient will go into congestive heart failure, furosemide can be given to keep the urine output approximately equal to the saline infusion rate.

The question of why therapy with fluid and diuretics does not cause the same problem that is being treated may arise. First, the IV fluid has no free H_2O and is in fact hypertonic compared to the patient's serum (0.9% saline = 154 mEq/L Na and has a tonicity of 308). Second, care is taken so that the dose of furosemide will not cause volume depletion, so the patient maintains good delivery of salt and H_2O to the distal nephron. Thirdly, although the furosemide does block the diluting sites of the thick ascending limb of Henle, the diluting sites of the distal tubule (those inhibited by thiazides) are functional. Once the thiazide effect wears off, maximally dilute urine can be made. Finally, by blocking the solute extraction in the thick ascending limb, the medullary tonicity falls, so even if ADH is present there is less osmotic gradient to pull H_2O from the dilute urine that is passing through the collecting ducts. The solute removed in the distal convoluted tubule does not contribute to the medullary tonicity, so thiazides do not reduce the medullary hypertonicity.

3. What advice would you give her to avoid this problem in the future?

In the future, Miss Caishun probably should not take thiazide or thiazide-like drugs including thiazide derivatives, metolazone, or indapamide; however, she could be treated with loop-active diuretics with relative safety.

CASE STUDY 4

Hyponatremia Associated with Hypopituitarism

John Bell, a patient with known anterior pituitary insufficiency secondary to Hand-Schuller-Christian disease, was involved in a motor vehicle accident. In the accident he sustained a head injury that resulted in a severe concussion. After two days in a comatose state, the patient began to recover, but then had a neurologic relapse, with increasing confusion and a decreasing level of consciousness. His only therapy at this time was 0.45% saline at 125 cc/h. At this point reevaluation reveals a blood pressure of 130/80 mmHg without significant orthostatic change; pulse 80 and regular, and respiration 16. Physical exam did not give evidence for volume overload or volume depletion.

LABORATORY DATA

Na 116 mEq/L	BUN 15 mg/dL	Plasma osm 249 mOsm/kg
K 3.9 mEq/L	Creatinine 1.1 mg/dL	Urinary osm 690 mOsm/kg
Cl 75 mEq/L	Glucose 135 mg/dL	Urinary Na 48 mEq/L
CO_2 28 mEq/L		

Question 1. Explain the role of pre-existing medical problems in the pathophysiology of hyponatremia in this patient.

Question 2. Which iatrogenic factors probably contributed to the hyponatremia?

Question 3. An eager medical student wanting to impress the attending in the morning performed a test to prove the diagnosis. What might he have done?

---

1. Explain the role of pre-existing medical problems in the pathophysiology of hyponatremia in this patient.

This patient's physical examination and laboratory studies all suggest that the hyponatremia falls into the euvolemic category. The known history of anterior pituitary insufficiency suggests that he could have glucocorticoid insufficiency. The cortisol deficiency causes a failure to suppress ADH release despite hypotonicity. The ADH blocks the kidney's ability to clear free H_2O by making the distal collecting ducts H_2O permeable. The evidence indicates that he was getting intravenous fluid containing free H_2O. This is significant because even with an elevated ADH, hyponatremia only develops if H_2O intake exceeds H_2O excretion.

2. Which iatrogenic factors probably contributed to the hyponatremia?

Failure to give glucocorticoids was one of the iatrogenic causes of his hyponatremia. The other was giving too much free H_2O in the intravenous fluid. Since hyponatremia is the result of an imbalance of H_2O intake and output, if less free water had been given then the hyponatremia would not have developed.

3. An eager medical student wanting to impress the attending in the morning performed a test to prove diagnosis. What might he have done?

The etiology of the hyponatremia is glucocorticoid deficiency, so measuring a serum cortisol level would confirm the diagnosis. Unfortunately, most labs do not run cortisol levels overnight so an alternate test needed to be devised.

The student realized that once glucocorticoids are given the ADH will be suppressed, and the patient will have a free-H_2O diuresis. By measuring the plasma and urine osmolality both before and after glucocorticoid administration, he should be able to prove his diagnosis. The urinary osmolality after glucocorticoids will be low (<50 mOsm/kg), which is consistent with a free-H_2O diuresis.

CASE STUDY 5

Hyponatremia Associated with Tumor-SIADH

Cy Adhze, a 54-year-old man, was brought into the emergency room because of a grand mal seizure. He had previously been diagnosed as having small cell carcinoma of the lung. He had not been on any medication recently and has not had any chemotherapy.

Physical examination showed the patient was in a post-ictal state, with blood pressure of 138/86 mmHg, and a pulse of 76 without orthostatic changes. The body temperature was 37°. The patient's neck was supple, with no Kernig or Brudzinski signs. Neck veins were visible 3 cm above the angle of Louis. Chest exam showed dullness over the right lung field base.

LABORATORY DATA

Na 105 mEq/L	BUN 5 mg/dL	Urinary Na 90 mEq/kg
K 4.0 mEq/L	Creatinine 1.0 mg/dL	Urinary K 64 mEq/kg
Cl 70 mEq/L	Glucose 85 mg/dL	U Urea nitrogen 150 mg/dL
CO_2 25 mEq/L		

Question 1. What is the differential diagnosis for this patient's hyponatremia?

Question 2. Calculate the free H_2O excess assuming a body weight of 60 kg.

Question 3. How would you manage this case?

Question 4. If 0.45% saline at 250 mL had been infusing during the 4 hours that the patient was in the emergency room, how much would this have corrected the electrolyte disturbance? For this calculation assume that urine output equaled intravenous fluid infusion rate, and that the spot urine electrolytes are representative of his subsequent urine.

---

1. What is the differential diagnosis for this patient's hyponatremia?

On clinical examination the patient is euvolemic. The urine osmolality is calculated as

$$\text{Urine osmolality} = 2 \times (\text{urinary Na}^+ + \text{urinary K}^+) + \text{urine urea nitrogen}/2.8$$
$$= 2 \times (90 + 64) + 150/2.8 \quad \text{(Eq. 2-18)}$$
$$= 362 \text{ mOsm/kg}$$

Urine osmolality should be less than serum osmolality when the serum tonicity is low. In this case the urine osmolality is inappropriately elevated, which is consistent with an inappropriately elevated serum ADH level. Mr. Adhze has many possible causes for SIADH, including a pulmonary process with the small cell carcinoma, and the tumor, which could release ADH. He is not receiving any new medications known to cause SIADH, and by history has not received any chemotherapeutic agent associated with SIADH. We are not told if Mr. Adhze has had nausea or vomiting, both of which can cause ADH release.

2. Calculate the free H_2O excess assuming a body weight of 60 kg.

$$H_2O \text{ excess} = 60 \text{ kg} \times 0.6 \times (1 - 105/140) = 9 \text{ liters} \qquad \text{(Eq. 2-19)}$$

3. How would you manage this case?

The management of profound hyponatremia is still controversial. On one hand, there are risks to not treating (including recurrent seizures); on the other hand, rapid changes in tonicity can lead to possible structural neurologic damage. In this case hyponatremia is causing significant morbidity. A more aggressive intervention, namely 3% saline infusion, is warranted. The goal of 3% saline infusion is to assure correction of the serum tonicity, in a controlled manner. The initial management should aim to correct the serum Na by about 5 mEq/L over 2 to 3 hours. To calculate the infusion rate, first determine the Na deficit. The Na deficit equals the rise in Na desired times the effective volume of distribution of Na. Total body water (TBW) is used as the effective volume of distribution, because TBW is the "space" influenced by Na even though Na is restricted to the extracellular space. This is because Na exerts a tonic action that shifts water from the intracellular to the extracellular space, and thereby influences the solute concentration in all fluid spaces.

$$
\begin{aligned}
Na^+ \text{ deficit} &= 5 \text{ mEq/L} \times TBW \\
&= 5 \times (60 \times .6) \qquad \text{(Eq. 2-20)} \\
&= 180 \text{ mEq}
\end{aligned}
$$

Three percent saline is 513 mEq/L (remember 0.9% saline = 154 mEq/L); therefore, approximately 350 mL of 3% saline needs to be infused over 2 to 3 hours. During this period, serum Na needs to be checked frequently, since these calculations were based on an assumption of no insensible H_2O losses. This assumption is only a crude approximation, since the patient will continue to lose Na and H_2O through the usual processes. Also, Cy Adhze needs to be carefully monitored for signs of heart failure, since the hypertonic saline will draw intracellular water into the vascular space and expand the intravascular volume. Once the serum Na reaches approximately 110 mEq/L, the hypertonic saline should be stopped. The remainder of the correction to a level of 130 mEq/L should proceed at approximately 0.5 mEq/L/h using saline and furosemide, or by free-H_2O restriction depending on the clinical setting.

4. If 0.45% saline at 250 mL/h had been infused during the 4 hours that the patient was in the emergency room, how much would this have corrected the electrolyte imbalance?

From the urine electrolytes we can calculate the H_2O and electrolyte losses. During the emergency room stay the patient received 1 L of 0.45% saline and excreted 1 L of urine. The electrolyte concentration of the urine is 154 mEq/L (urinary Na + urinary K = 90 + 64 = 154). The electrolyte concentration of intravenous fluid is 77 mEq/L. Therefore over the four hours, the patient had a net gain of 500 mL ($1 L \times 77/154 = 500$) of H_2O. In terms of serum Na, this would have the following effect:

$$\text{serum Na}^+ = 60 \times 0.6 \times 120/(60 \times 0.6 + 0.5) = 118 \text{ mEq/L} \qquad \text{(Eq. 2-21)}$$

The infusion of 0.45% saline caused a fall in serum Na, because the urine is more electrolyte rich than the intravenous fluid. It is important to appreciate the value of urinary electrolytes when considering intravenous fluid orders in these cases.

The above calculations assumed that Na^+ was distributed throughout the TBW (i.e., Na^+ deficit = $Na^+ \times$ TBW). Obviously, the ICF (i.e., two-thirds of the TBW) has almost no Na^+, but its principal cation is K^+. For the purposes of determining Na^+ balance, Na^+ can be considered equal to K^+ because for every Na^+ extracellular there needs to be a K^+ intracellular to maintain osmotic balance across the cell membrane. So, in the calculations of urine electrolyte loss, urinary Na^+ + urinary K^+ is compared to Na^+ infusion. Isotope dilution studies have proven that

$$\text{Serum Na}^+ = \frac{\text{Total body Na}^+ + \text{Total body K}^+}{\text{Total body water}} \qquad \text{(Eq. 2-22)}$$

Thus, you must always add the total cation ($Na^+ + K^+$) content of urine and divide it by urine volume to determine whether a patient's urine output is more or less dilute than the infusate. This is a key guide to future therapy of hyponatremic patients.

CASE STUDY 6

Hyponatremia Associated with Congestive Heart Failure

P. Flow, a 52-year-old male with a past history of hypertension and a recent massive anterior wall myocardial infarction, presented to the emergency room complaining of shortness of breath. He stated that the shortness of breath had been gradually worsening over the past week, concomitant with the development of pedal edema. He denied any recent anginal pain, but reported a slow rise in his weight from 60 to 75 kg. He admitted to not complying with his low sodium diet. His only outpatient medicine was transdermal nitroglycerin. On a recent clinic visit he had a Na level of 135 mEq/L and a creatinine level of 1.5 mg/dL.

His physical examination revealed a weight of 75 kg, blood pressure of 110/70 mmHg, and heart rate of 100 without orthostatic changes. His neck veins distended to 12 cm at a 45-degree elevation. Lung examination revealed rales $\frac{1}{3}$ up, bilaterally. Cardiac exam revealed soft S_3. The rectal exam was negative for blood. Extremities showed 2+ pitting edema to the knees.

LABORATORY DATA

Na 128 mEq/L	BUN 70 mg/dL
K 4.0 mEq/L	Creatinine 2.0 mg/dL
Cl 89 mEq/L	Glucose 125 mg/dL
CO_2 30 mEq/L	serum Osm (measured) 295 mOsm/kg

ECG without change from baseline

Question 1. Given the low serum Na with a high normal serum osmolality, could this be factitious hyponatremia?

Question 2. What is the patient's volume (sodium) status?

Question 3. What is the etiology of the hyponatremia?

Question 4. How would you manage this patient's electrolyte disorder while he is in the hospital?

Question 5. What discharge instructions would you give the patient to try to prevent a recurrence?

---

1. Given the low serum Na with high normal serum osmolality, could this be factitious hyponatremia?

Factitious hyponatremia occurs when effective solutes are added to the ECF. These solutes draw H_2O from the ICF, which dilutes the Na in the ECF. In factitious hyponatremia, the osmolality is normal-to-high due to the addition of an effective osmol. In this case the measured osmolality is normal, but this is due to the presence of an ineffective osmol, urea. The *tonicity* of Mr. Flow is markedly reduced in spite of the normal serum osmolality. The tonicity can be calculated as follows

$$\text{Tonicity} = 2 \times Na^+ + \text{glucose}/18$$
$$= 256 + 8 \qquad \text{(Eq. 2-23)}$$
$$= 264$$

2. What is the patient's volume (sodium) status?

This patient is both volume and Na overloaded as evidenced by the peripheral edema and signs of heart failure, including rales and an elevated CVP. In spite of the Na overload, he is hyponatremic.

3. What is the etiology of the hyponatremia?

The patient falls into the clinical category of volume-overload hyponatremia. The underlying cause of the hyponatremia is that H_2O intake exceeded renal free-H_2O clearance.

The renal insufficiency reduces his H_2O excretory capacity, but this is not the primary cause of the reduced free-H_2O clearance. The elevated serum creatinine is consistent with a reduced GFR. The creatinine clearance, which is an estimation of the GFR, can be calculated using the Cockroft-Gault formula. This formula takes into account body size, age, and gender as three independent variables in serum creatinine levels. The Cockroft-Gault formula is written as

$$\text{CrCl (est)} = \frac{140 - \text{age}}{\text{serum Cr}} \times \frac{\text{Wt in kg}}{70} \times (0.85 \text{ if female; } 1.0 \text{ if male}) \qquad \text{(Eq. 2-24)}$$

For Mr. Flow this gives an estimated creatinine clearance of 45 mL/min.

As can be seen from Figure 2-1, if this were the only perturbation in the H_2O clearance mechanism, then the patient could still clear large quantities of H_2O, approximately 8 to 10 L/day.

Hyponatremia is one of the most frequent electrolyte abnormalities in heart failure. The decreased cardiac output leads directly to a reduction in renal blood flow (kidneys perceive a decreased EABV). The decreased EABV causes an increased proximal urine reabsorption, which reduces the quantity of free H_2O that can be cleared by the kidneys. The decreased renal blood flow also stimulates renin release which ultimately results in an elevated AII level. The elevated AII leads to impaired H_2O clearance by (1) stimulating thirst and therefore increasing H_2O intake, and (2) stimulating vasopressin release from the pituitary, which makes the collecting ducts permeable to H_2O; this impairs excretion of a dilute urine.

4. How would you manage this patient's electrolyte disorder while he is in the hospital?

The patient's primary clinical problem is heart failure and not hyponatremia. The patient does not have symptoms related to his reduced tonicity, but does have symptoms of volume overload. Treatment should be tailored to the heart failure; at the same time, this will help correct the disturbance in the H_2O excretory mechanism.

Diuresis with furosemide typically results in urine with a urine Na and K of approximately 75. Therefore, about half of all urine output will be free H_2O, which will help correct the hyponatremia.

Vasodilating agents should improve cardiac output which, in turn, will improve renal blood flow. The increased renal blood flow will reduce proximal urinary reabsorption, leading to increased distal delivery of urine. This urine then potentially can be diluted in the thick ascending limb and subsequently excreted as a dilute (free H_2O rich) urine. If an ACE inhibitor is used as the vasodilating agent, this will inhibit AII production, which will help with the problems mentioned in answer 3 of this case.

While the above therapies are being instituted, it is important to strictly limit the patient's H_2O intake (both p.o. fluids and hyponatremic intravenous fluids).

5. What discharge instructions would you give the patient to try to prevent a recurrence?

As an outpatient, Mr. Flow must limit his Na intake (to prevent heart failure), and limit his H_2O intake (to prevent hyponatremia). The degree of limitation necessary will depend on his cardiac output after therapeutic interventions.

CASE STUDY 7

Hyponatremia Secondary to Exogenous ADH Administration

Lotte Acqua, a 45-year-old woman with a long history of non-A, non-B hepatitis, was brought to the emergency room complaining of hematemesis, which started 15 minutes before presentation. Blood samples were drawn, and she was admitted to the intensive care unit. On presentation to the ICU she was found to be hypotensive and was stabilized with 4 units of packed red blood cells and 2 liters of 0.9% saline. The laboratory results on the blood drawn in the emergency room were remarkable for a Na level of 132 mEq/L, glucose of 100 mg/dL, albumin 2.0 mg/dL, PT 14.0 sec, TB 4.5 mg/dL, BUN 5 mg/dL, and creatinine of 1.0 mg/dL. During her first hospital day, the GI bleeding recurred. Endoscopy revealed esophageal varices. To control the bleeding a pitressin infusion was initiated.

On the second hospital day Ms. Acqua's serum Na fell to 130 mEq/L. All intravenous fluids were changed to 0.9% saline and she was made NPO. Her intake and output were equal at 2500 ml.

Her physical examination showed weight of 50 kg, blood pressure of 110/70 mmHg, and heart rate 80 without orthostatic changes. Her skin was jaundiced with telangiectases, neck with JVD to 3 cm at 45 degrees, and lungs clear to auscultation. Cardiac exam revealed no S_3, abdominal exam revealed a fluid wave, and back exam revealed 2 + presacral edema. The neurologic exam showed her to be alert and oriented to person, place, and time, with no asterixis.

LABORATORY DATA

Third Day

Na 129 mEq/L CO_2 30 mEq/L
K 4.0 mEq/L   serum osm 270 mOsm/kg
Cl 85 mEq/L

A spot urine was trace protein on dipstick and urine electrolytes were

Urine Na 125 mEq/L   Urine K 50 mEq/L   Urine osm 750 mOsm/kg

---

Question 1. Why did the patient have a serum Na level of 132 mEq/L on admission?
Question 2. Why did her Na continue to fall between the second and third hospital day despite her not drinking H_2O?
Question 3. How would you try to correct her hyponatremia and manage her fluids?

---

1. Why did the patient have a serum Na level of 132 mEq/L on admission?

Evaluating the patient's clinical status is very helpful in determining the etiology of the hyponatremia. She presumably was not hypovolemic before the GI bleed. Ms. Acqua's physical exam is consistent with total body sodium overload as judged by the presacral edema and ascites. She has a history of significant liver disease and manifests the sequela of cirrhosis, including portal hypertension with varices, ascites, hypoalbuminemia, hyperbilirubinemia, and a coagulopathy. Patients with severe liver disease often have a decreased EABV despite total body Na overload. This decreased EABV is secondary to peripheral vasodilation, hypoalbuminemia, and splanchnic venous pooling with ascites formation. The decreased EABV causes an increased proximal tubular reabsorption of Na and, thus, H_2O retention. The decreased EABV also stimulates ADH release. Her hyponatremia developed because she consumed more H_2O than her kidneys could excrete.

2. Why did her Na continue to fall between the second and third hospital day, in spite of her not drinking H_2O?

Her urine electrolyte concentration is greater than the electrolyte concentration of the intravenous fluid (negative free-H_2O clearance). In essence Ms. Acqua's kidneys are generating free H_2O from the 0.9% saline she receives. This can be viewed quantitatively as follows

	Urine	Intravenous fluid
H_2O	2500 mL	2500 mL
Na + K	438 mEq	385 mEq

Therefore, during the second hospital day her H_2O volume remained constant, but her Na content fell by 53 mEq. This means that her serum Na should fall by

$$\text{serum Na}^+ = \frac{(45 \times 0.6 \times 130) - 53}{45 \times 0.6} = 128 \qquad \text{(Eq. 2-25)}$$

The difference between the calculated and measured serum Na probably reflects insensible H_2O loss.

Ms. Acqua's worsening hyponatremia should be expected, since she had a negative urinary free-H_2O clearance. Patients develop negative free-H_2O clearances when they have intact renal concentrating mechanisms. In this patient, maximally concentrated urine exists because she is in a high ADH state—pitressin is an ADH analogue.

3. How would you try to correct her hyponatremia and manage her fluids?

As long as Ms. Acqua is on the pitressin infusion she will be H_2O retentive. To prevent worsening hyponatremia, the intravenous fluid can be made more hypertonic or her renal concentrating mechanism can be blocked. Hypertonic fluids are generally not used, because they will worsen a patient's baseline volume overload. Furosemide is an effective agent for blunting her renal concentrating ability. If she receives furosemide, her intravascular volume status must be carefully monitored to prevent further reduction of her EABV.

FURTHER READINGS

Abramow M, Cogan E: Clinical aspects and pathophysiology of diuretic-induced hyponatremia. Adv Nephrol 13:1, 1984

Dargie HJ: Interrelation of electrolytes and renin-angiotensin system in congestive heart failure. Am J Cardiol 65:28E, 1990

DeFronzo RA, Goldberg M, Agus A: Normal diluting capacity in hyponatremic patients: reset osmostat or a variant of inappropriate antidiuretic hormone secretion. Ann Intern Med 84:538, 1976

Oelker W: Hyponatremia and inappropriate secretion of vasopressin (antidiuretic hormone) in patients with hypopituitarism. N Engl J Med 321(8):492, 1989

Papadakis MA, Fraser CL, Arieff AI: Hyponatremia in patients with cirrhosis. Quart J Med 76:675, 1990

Stern RH: Treating hyponatremia: what is all the controversy about? Ann Intern Med 113(6):417, 1990

Sterns RH: The treatment of hyponatremia: unsafe at any speed? Nephrol Let 6(1):1, 1989

Weisberg LS: Pseudohyponatremia: a reappraisal. Am J Med 86:315, 1989

3

Hypernatremia

Gail Morrison

Hypernatremia is defined as a serum sodium concentration greater than 145 mEq/L. Two-thirds of total body water (TBW) is distributed to the intracellular fluid compartment (ICF) and one-third to the extracellular fluid compartment (ECF). The ECF is composed of the plasma compartment (one-fourth) and the interstitial compartment (three-fourths). Cell membranes separating these compartments are freely permeable to water and to solutes identified as *permeant* or *non-effective* osmoles (Fig. 3-1). Sodium, with its anion, chloride, or biocarbonate is confined to the ECF compartment.

OSMOLES

Effective (Nonpermeant) Osmoles

Solutes that do not passively cross the cell membrane exert an osmotic pressure across that cell membrane and are called effective osmoles. Sodium, chloride, and bicarbonate, glucose and special solutes used in specific clinical situations (e.g. mannitol, glycerol, and sorbitol) are all effective osmoles restricted to the ECF compartment. An increase in their concentration in the ECF compartment will increase the osmotic pressure in the ECF and result in a shift of water from the ICF to the ECF. Potassium, magnesium, phosphates, sulfates, and proteins are effective osmoles restricted to the ICF. An increase in their concentration in the ICF will increase the osmotic pressure in the ICF and result in an opposite shift of water, from the ECF to the ICF.

Consequence of Effective Osmoles

Distribution of TBW between the ECF and ICF is determined by the quantity of osmotically active solutes (i.e., quantity of effective osmoles) in each compartment. Normally, the ICF contains two-thirds and the ECF contains one-third of the body's osmotically active solutes. As a result, two-thirds of TBW is located in the ICF; one-third of TBW is located in the ECF (Fig. 3-2). However, because all cell membranes are freely permeable to water, the ECF osmolality

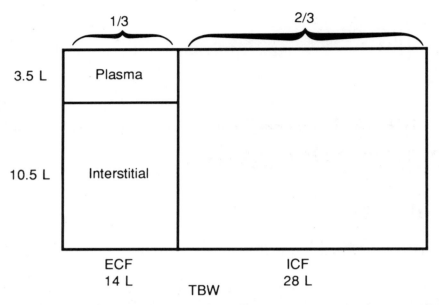

Fig. 3-1. Body fluid compartments. Total body H_2O (TBW) accounts for 60% of lean body mass in a 70 kg man (42 L). Two-thirds of TBW (28 L) is located in the ICF and one-third (14 L) is located in the ECF. One-fourth of the ECF (3.5 L) is intravascular; three-fourths (10.5) of ECF is interstitial.

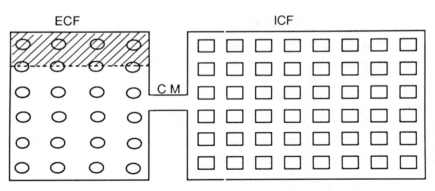

Fig. 3-2. Distribution of H_2O and solute. The larger square (right) represents the ICF compartment and the smaller square (left) represents the ECF compartment. The bridge connecting the two compartments represents the cell membranes (CM). The volumes of the two compartments are represented by the areas of the outer squares. The small symbols (open squares, open circles) represent intracellular solutes (largely K salts) and extracellular solutes (largely Na salts), respectively. The number of small symbols represents the solute content of each compartment, and the density of symbols represents the solute concentration (osmolality) of the compartment. (See text for details.) (From Feig PU, McCurdy DK: The hypertonic state. N Engl J Med 297:1444, 1977, with permission.)

is equal to the ICF osmolality. The volumes of the two compartments then reflect their respective "effective" solute contents.

Ineffective (Permeant) Osmoles

Solutes, which, like water, passively cross the cell membrane, do not exert an osmotic pressure across the cell membrane because they distribute throughout TBW. These solutes are ineffective or permeant osmoles. If present, they will increase the solute concentration and thus, osmolality throughout TBW. These solutes will not cause water to shift from the ECF to the ICF or from the ICF to the ECF. Clinically, blood urea nitrogen (BUN) and ethanol are the primary ineffective or permeant osmoles encountered.

PLASMA OSMOLALITY VERSUS PLASMA TONICITY

Plasma Osmolality (Posm)

By measuring the freezing point depression of a plasma sample one can determine the amount of both effective and noneffective osmoles in that sample. This measurement, the plasma osmolality (Posm), reflects the osmolality throughout TBW. The Posm can be calculated:

$$\text{Posm} = 2 \, (\text{Na}) \, \text{mEq/L} + \frac{\text{glucose mg/dL}}{18} + \frac{\text{BUN mg/dL}}{2.8} + \frac{\text{X mg/dL}}{\text{mol wt/10}} \qquad \text{(Eq. 3-1)}$$

Where X = ethanol mol wt 46
            mannitol mol wt 180
            sorbitol mol wt 180
            glycerol mol wt 9

mol wt = molecular weight

Normal range for plasma osm is 280 to 295 mOsm/kg. An estimated Posm = 2 (Na) + 10 since the major solute contributing to Posm is sodium (Na) plus its accompanying anion, either chloride or bicarbonate. Glucose and urea normally contribute less than 10 mOsm/kg. Of importance, it is not routine to measure the specific concentration of substances listed under "X". Therefore, a significant discrepancy between the measured and calculated Posm (i.e., a difference of >10 mOsm/kg) means there is an unmeasured solute present, "X", in addition to Na, glucose, and BUN.

Plasma Tonicity

This is a term used to identify effective plasma osmolality. It can not be measured, but can be calculated using the concentration measurements of substances that generate an osmotic pressure across the cell membrane (i.e., effective osmoles). The formula to calculate plasma tonicity (effective Posm) is:

$$\text{Plasma Tonicity} = 2 \, (\text{Na}^+) \, \text{mEq/L} + \frac{\text{glucose mg/dL}}{18} + \frac{\text{X mg/dL}}{\text{mol wt/10}} \qquad \text{(Eq. 3-2)}$$

Where X *can* be sorbitol, mannitol, or glycerol but *not* ethanol or BUN, which are ineffective osmoles.

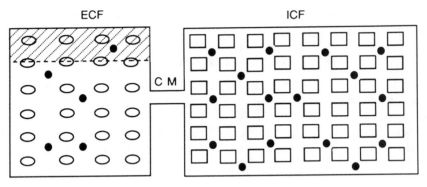

Fig. 3-3. Hyperosmolality without hypertonicity (permeant solute gain). An ineffective (permeant) solute, such as urea or ethanol (small solid circles), diffuses across all cell membranes (CM); it therefore distributes throughout TBW. Thus, permeant solutes do not exert an osmotic force for H_2O movement from one compartment to another, and there is no change in the volumes of the ECF or ICF. Hyperosmolality, but not hypertonicity, is the result of addition of a permeant solute.

The normal range for plasma tonicity is 270 to 285 mOsm/kg. Estimated plasma tonicity is 2 (Na).

HYPEROSMOLALITY WITHOUT HYPERTONICITY

Two clinical conditions, azotemia and ethanol ingestion, are associated with an increase in ineffective osmoles: substances that increase the solute concentration throughout TBW without altering the osmotic pressure across the cell membrane. An increase in BUN (azotemia) or the presence of ethanol will increase the Posm of both the ECF and ICF. Because permeant solutes distribute throughout TBW, there are *no* shifts of water between the ECF and ICF compartments (Fig. 3-3).

HYPERTONICITY

As the calculated formula for plasma tonicity indicates (Eq. 3-2), hypertonicity will be most frequently associated with conditions that cause hypernatremia and hyperglycemia. (In special clinical circumstances glycerol, mannitol, or sorbitol may cause hypertonicity.) Hypertonicity always has two features:

- ↑ Posm and an ↑ effective Posm as a result of an increase in the concentration of effective solutes.
- ICF contraction because the ↑ effective Posm will cause water to shift from the ICF to the ECF until the osmolalities of both compartments are once again equal.

CONSEQUENCES OF ECF HYPERTONICITY

Cellular Dehydration

ECF hypertonicity causes water to shift from the ICF to the ECF until the Posm ECF = Posm ICF. The result is *cellular dehydration* (contraction of the ICF). Of particular concern, brain cells, in response to cellular dehydration, generate "idiogenic osmoles" that raise the intracellular effective Posm and cause water to shift intracellularly to re-establish normal brain cell volume.

The rapidity of the development of idiogenic osmoles is dependent on the specific solute causing ECF hypertonicity.

Condition	Time for normalization of brain cell volume	Idiogenic Osmoles
Hypernatremia	1 week	Na, Amino acids
Hyperglycemia	4–6 hours	Na;? other undetermined osmoles
Sorbitol, mannitol, glycerol	?	?

Although idiogenic osmoles may appear to protect the brain cells from long term cellular dehydration, it is disturbing to find that the substance frequently identified as an idiogenic osmole is Na. Most of the time, an increase in the intracellular concentration of Na generally indicates cell damage and impairment of the Na^+K^+-ATPase pump. Of even more concern, the rapidity of the removal of these idiogenic osmoles is unknown. Thus, a consequence of rapid correction of hypertonicity with free water, before idiogenic osmoles disappear, is a very significant complication, cerebral edema.

Clinical Neurologic Consequences

Brain cell dehydration causes neurologic complications including fatigue, lethargy, and changes in mental status such as confusion and mental obtundation. The more hypertonic the ECF fluids are, the more severe are the neurological symptoms. Seizures, coma, and even death can occur. The very young (infants) are particularly susceptible to neurologic complications and long-term neurologic sequelae because the fragility of their blood vessels makes them prone to develop subdural hemorrhages and cerebral bleeding with hypertonic conditions. On the other hand, most adults do not have significant complications like seizures or coma until the Na concentration approaches 170 mEq/L.

PATHOGENESIS OF HYPERNATREMIA

Hypernatremia may result from three separate pathologic conditions. First, conditions associated with a loss of electrolyte-free fluids (loss of pure water). Second are conditions associated with a gain of a solute restricted to the ECF compartment. Finally, conditions associated with the loss of hypotonic fluids (fluids containing more water than sodium) can cause hypernatremia. The pathophysiologic findings associated with hypernatremia are increased Posm, increased effective Posm (Plasma tonicity), and ICF Contraction. There are two important physiologic responses to hypernatremia: (1) increased serum Na will increase Posm and effective Posm and stimulate the release of ADH from the posterior pituitary gland. ADH, by its action on the distal tubule and collecting duct of the nephron, will result in increased reabsorption of "free" water.

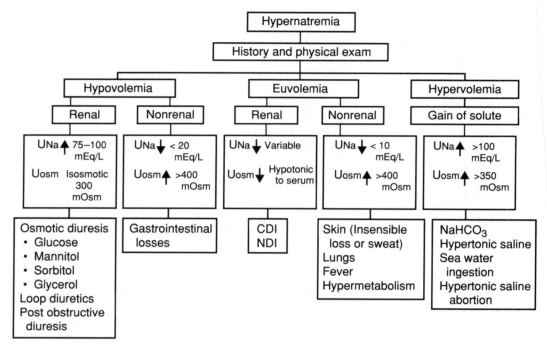

Fig. 3-4. Pathogenesis of hypernatremia.

A Uosm greater than 400 mOsm/kg indicates the presence and effect of ADH. (2) Increased serum Na should stimulate the brain's thirst center and result in an individual increasing his intake of water.

APPROACH TO HYPERNATREMIA

The patient's history often suggests conditions associated with the development of hyponatremia, but since many individuals with hypernatremia will have significant mental status changes, an accurate history may be impossible to obtain. The physical exam may be particularly helpful if one can assess whether the individual is euvolemic, hypervolemic, or hypovolemic. Certain laboratory data, including electrolytes, BUN, creatinine, glucose, Posm, calculated effective Posm, urinary osmolality (Uosm) and urinary electrolytes—especially UNa, may further determine the etiology for the hypernatremia (Fig. 3-4).

GENERAL READINGS

Arieff AI: Osmotic failure: physiology and strategies for treatment. Hosp Pract 23:173, 1988
Rose BD: New approach to disturbances in plasma sodium concentration. Am J Med 81:1033, 1986
Feig PU, McCurdy DK: The hypertonic state. N Engl J Med 297:1444, 1977
Feig PU: Hypernatremia and hypertonic syndromes. Med Clin North Am 65:271, 1981
Mathisen O: Mechanisms of osmotic diuresis. Kidney Int 19:431, 1981

CASE STUDY 1

Hypernatremia Secondary to Dehydration

Miss Daisy, a 79-year-old woman who resides in a nursing home, was brought to the hospital because of decreased mental acuity. She had been doing well until she developed a fever associated with an upper respiratory tract infection. She ate poorly and over 3 days became less responsive. She had been treated with antibiotics but not intravenous fluids. Her physical examination showed her to be a disoriented and obtunded elderly woman. Her blood pressure was 108/78; pulse 96; respiration 20; temperature 102.4°. Her weight on admission was 50 kg. Skin had poor turgor, decreased axillary seat, her chest was clear and heart had regular rhythm, with no murmurs or gallops. The abdomen was without masses and extremities without edema.

LABORATORY DATA

Na 167 mEq/L	BUN 26 mg/dL	Hbg 18.1 gm/dL
K 4.3 mEq/L	Creatinine 1.0 mg/dL	Hct 44%
Cl 120 mEq/L	Glucose 100 mg/dL	
HCO_3 29 mEq/L		

Urinalysis: negative dipstick S.G. 1.022
microscopic exam: negative

Question 1. How does the history, physical exam, and laboratory data help in identifying the pathophysiologic mechanism responsible for the development of hypernatremia?

Question 2. How does her ECF and ICF compartments compare to those found in a normal individual?

Question 3. What other conditions associated with loss of electrolyte-free fluids cause hypernatremia?

Question 4. Calculate her free-H_2O deficit.

Question 5. How would you manage her hypernatremia?

---

1. How does the history, physical exam, and laboratory data help in identifying the pathophysiologic mechanism responsible for the development of hypernatremia?

In the patient's history, the presence of conditions that predispose to a loss of electrolyte-free water and a deficit in water intake are important. Fever causes an increase in *insensible losses*. For each 1°F increase in body temperature over 100°F, an individual loses 1000 ml of additional electrolyte free fluid as sweat. Normally, insensible loss averages 500 mL/day. Disorientation, mental obtundation, and changes in an individual's mental status are often associated with a diminished thirst perception and/or decreased ability to access water (an inability to either physically obtain it or to drink it).

To become hypernatremic an individual must have a condition that predisposes her to lose free water (i.e., fever) and a loss of thirst perception and/or access to water. As the serum Na concentration rises to the upper limits of normal (145 mEq/L) with loss of electrolyte-free water, the individual should be "driven" by her thirst center to drink adequate quantities of water to maintain the serum Na concentration at 145 mEq/L or less.

The patient's physical exam and laboratory data reveal

Hypernatremia without evidence of hypotension or shock;

Disorientation and obtundation suggesting CNS alterations;

Fever to 102.4°F, causing ongoing increased insensible water losses (e.g., sweat);

Poor skin turgor, decreased axillary sweat despite fever and dry mucous membranes in association with a normal blood pressure and pulse suggests euvolemia and cellular dehydration;

Hypernatremia (167 mEq/L) indicates hyperosmolality (Posm of 344 mOsm/kg) and hypertonicity (effective Posm 339 mOsm/kg);

Urinalysis reveals a concentrated urine with a specific gravity of 1.022 suggesting both the presence and effect of ADH;

Urine osmolality is generally twice that of plasma (a concentrated urine) for a nonrenal cause for free water loss.

According to the algorithm (Fig. 3-4), the history, physical exam, and lab data are consistent with a loss of electrolyte free water and a nonrenal cause for free water loss (e.g., sweating)—associated with an inability to access free water.

2. How do her ECF and ICF compartments compare with those found in a normal individual (Fig. 3-2).

Electrolyte free water is lost from TBW in the same proportion as it is normally found. As Figure 3-5 indicates, two-thirds of these losses occur from the ICF and one-third from the ECF.

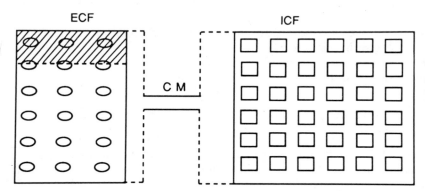

Fig. 3-5. Hypertonicity due to pure H_2O loss. Pure H_2O deficit is shared proportionally by all body fluid compartments, according to the effective solute content of each compartment. Therefore, both the ECF and the ICF will contract: two-thirds of the deficit will be derived from the ICF and one-third from the ECF. Only one-twelfth of the total H_2O loss will be derived from the intravascular compartment. (The dotted lines indicate the normal volumes of the body fluid compartments.) The total amount of solute in each compartment remains constant, but the solute concentration (osmolality) increases. (CM, cell membranes.)

Loss of electrolyte-free water concentrates all solutes in the ECF and the ICF. Since Na is the major solute in the ECF, there is an increase in the serum Na concentration, or hypernatremia.

Since the plasma compartment is only one-fourth of the ECF compartment, only one-twelfth of each liter of free water (80 mL) lost from TBW comes from the plasma compartment. Therefore, although there is a contraction of TBW, the major effect is on the ICF compartment. As a result, on the physical exam, there is generally evidence for euvolemia, with cellular dehydration (poor skin turgor, decreased axillary sweat, CNS disorientation).

The cells most affected by cellular dehydration are brain cells. Brain cell dehydration initially causes mental status changes and obtundation, but if severe can progress to seizures or coma. A significant consequence of hypertonicity is the accumulation of idiogenic osmoles within brain cells.

3. What other conditions associated with loss of electrolyte-free fluids cause hypernatremia?

Both renal and nonrenal conditions can cause loss of electrolyte-free fluids from the body. The Uosm and UNa can be helpful in differentiating between renal and nonrenal conditions.

Renal
Any disease or condition causing central (CDI) or nephrogenic (NDI) diabetes insipidus can cause hypernatremia if associated with a decreased thirst perception and/or decreased access to water. Both CDI and NDI tend to have increased volumes of urine with inappropriately low Uosm for the degree of serum hypertonicity. Remember, a serum sodium concentration greater than 145 mEq/L should stimulate the release of ADH, which should cause increased reabsorption of free water across the collecting duct of the nephron and result in a concentrated urine (increased Uosm or increased specific gravity with decreased urine volume).

Nonrenal
Other causes of electrolyte-free losses include hypermetabolic states, high ambient temperature (with increased sweating), and respiratory losses on a respirator. Conditions associated with these causes will have a urine showing the presence and effect of ADH.

4. Calculate her free-H_2O deficit.

To calculate the patient's free-H_2O deficit we need to know her weight (in kg) when she is not hypernatremic or at the present time (when she is hypernatremic).

The formula is

$$(2)(Na^+ \text{ mEq/L})(TBW)1 = 2 (Na^+ \text{ mEq/L})(TBW) \tag{Eq. 3-3}$$
$$\text{present} \quad \text{present} \quad \text{normal} \quad \text{normal}$$

We assume TBW = 60% of body wt (kg) (for a woman, use 50% because she has relatively more fat), that normal serum Na = 140 to 144 mEq/L, and that present weight (given) is 50 kg and present serum Na (given) is 167 mEq/L. There is no loss of Na for the body if the patient is euvolemic.

$$(2)(167) \times (0.5)(60) = (2)(140)(x)$$

$$\frac{167}{140} \times 30 = x \tag{Eq. 3-4}$$

$$35.7 \text{ liters} = x$$

Free-H_2O deficit = 35.7 − 30 = 5.7 L

5. How would you manage her hypernatremia?

Free-H_2O Repletion: Route
If mentally alert, oral ingestion is the preferred route. However, if disoriented or obtunded, intravenous administration of 5% D 5/w will be the recommended treatment.

Free-H_2O Repletion: Timing
Slow administration of H_2O, regardless of the route, is both recommended and desirable to prevent rapid correction of the hypernatremia, because if significant idiogenic osmoles have accumulated within brain cells, there is a high potential for developing cerebral edema with rapid infusion of H_2O.

Recommendations
One-half of calculated fluid losses repleted in first 24 hours
Remainder, repleted in next 24 to 48 hours
Remember to keep up with any ongoing losses so that further free-H_2O loss does not occur.
If the serum Na concentration continues to rise with repletion then you have not adequately assessed the ongoing free-H_2O losses correctly.

CASE STUDY 2

Hypernatremia Secondary to Hypertonic Solute Administration

Mr. Charles Bigheart, a 60-year-old man, had a cardiac arrest while in the emergency room after experiencing severe chest pain for 8 hours at home. He was immediately given CPR, which included a variety of drugs (epinephrine, calcium chloride, and sodium bicarbonate). He finally was resuscitated and brought to the ICU in stable condition. On physical examination the patient was intubated but responsive. His blood pressure was 150/100 mmHg; pulse 100; and temperature 99°F. His weight was 70 kg. Chest exam revealed diffuse rales, and heart showed S_3, S_4 gallop. His neck veins were distended. Abdomen was without masses, liver slightly enlarged, and extremities were without edema.

LABORATORY DATA

Na 161 mEq/L	BUN 18 mg/dL	Glucose 120
K 4.6 mEq/L	Creatinine 1.0 mg/dL	UNa 180 mEq/L
Cl 100 mEq/L		UK 50 mEq/L
HCO_3 37 mEq/L		

Urinanalysis: negative glucose, ketones, protein, blood.
Microscopic analysis: negative SG 1.021

Question 1. **How do the history, physical exam, and laboratory data help in identifying the pathophysiologic mechanism responsible for the development of hypernatremia?**

Question 2. How do his ECF and ICF compartments compare to those found in a normal individual?

Question 3. What other conditions associated with gain of effective osmoles cause hypernatremia?

Question 4. How would you manage his hypernatremia?

Question 5. Calculate the free-H_2O deficit.

---

1. **How do the history, physical exam, and laboratory data help in identifying the pathophysiologic mechanism responsible for the development of hypernatremia?**

The history is consistent with the ingestion or administration of a sodium-containing hypertonic solution. The patient received $NaHCO_3$ during a cardiac arrest. One ampule of $NaHCO_3$ contains 44 mEq of Na and 44 mEq of HCO_3 in 50 mL. A liter of this solution would have 1786 mEq or 1786 mOsm; making it a very hypertonic solution. (1 liter of normal saline has 150 mEq/L Na + 150 mEq/L Cl = 300 mOsm.)

The physical exam reveals a hypervolemic state: hypertension (BP 150/100), distended neck veins and evidence for CHF (rales and an S_3 gallop). Since he is on a respirator, it is not possible to accurately assess the degree to which the elevated sodium is affecting his mental status. With a sodium of 161 mEq/L, some alterations in his mental status would be expected.

Laboratory findings indicate:

Hypernatremia (Na 161 mEq/L)
Increased Posm = 2 (161) + 120/18 + 18/3 = 345 mOsm
Increased effective Posm = 2 (161) + 120/18 = 339 mOsm
Normal BUN consistent with hypervolemia
Increased urine volume from a sodium diuresis
Iso-hypertonic urine (Uosm > 300 mOsm) from the solute diuresis
UNa generally elevated indicating a saline diuresis (given: UNa = 180 mEq/L)

2. **How do his ECF and ICF compartments compare with those found in a normal individual (Fig. 3-2).**

Although $NaHCO_3$ was administered into the intravascular space (plasma compartment), it distributes immediately throughout the ECF compartment and raises the concentration of sodium and bicarbonate. Since Na is an effective osmole, the increased concentration of Na will raise the osmotic pressure across all cell membranes and cause intracellular dehydration (a shift of H_2O from the ICF to the ECF). As H_2O shifts into the ECF, there will be expansion of the ECF and contraction of the ICF until the ECF Posm = the ICF Posm. (See Fig. 3-6.) Clinically, this ECF expansion can present as pulmonary edema and/or CHF.

3. **What other conditions associated with gain of effective osmoles causes hypernatremia?**

Inadvertent administration of hypertonic saline solutions—3% or 5% NaCl having 500 mEq/L and 830 mEq/L, respectively—will result in hypernatremia. Saline abortions, which use hypertonic NaCl, can cause hypernatremia if the solution is inadvertently administered into the vascular

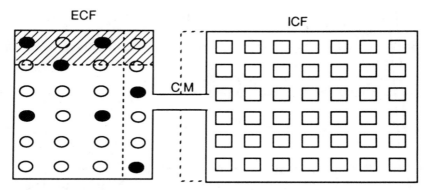

Fig. 3-6. Hypertonicity due to impermeant solute gain. The addition of an "effective" solute to the ECF expands the ECF compartment and contracts the ICF compartment as water moves from the ICF to the ECF in response to the osmotic gradient. The relative volumes of the two compartments change to reflect their present relative solute contents. Therefore, when the steady state (osmolal equilibrium) is reached, all body fluids are equally hypertonic. (CM, cell membranes.)

compartment and not the amniotic sac. Salt water drownings can, if there is significant ingestion of sea water, result in reabsorption of large amounts of NaCl.

4. How would you manage his hypernatremia?

Although one can calculate the amount of free H_2O necessary to lower the Na concentration to normal, administration of free H_2O is not the initial treatment of choice. As Figure 3-6 indicates, removal of Na as NaCl or $NaHCO_3$ is necessary to normalize ECF volume and to treat his CHF and pulmonary edema. With normal renal function, an individual can excrete a urine containing high concentrations of Na (in this case, 180 mEq/L) with an equal amount of an anion $(A-)$. Often times, following CPR, decreased cardiac function may cause renal insufficiency or failure, and then, dialysis or CAVH may need to be implemented. In many cases, a loop diuretic (e.g., furosemide) is given to augment urine flow. However, since these diuretics result in urine that loses both Na and H_2O, free-H_2O repletion must be instituted concurrent with diuretic administration to prevent a further rise in the serum Na concentration.

5. Calculate the free-H_2O deficit.

One can calculate the free-H_2O deficit at the time of presentation: Assume no loss of Na; only a shift of H_2O. Assume normal Na concentration $= 140 - 144$ mEq/L. If present weight is 50 kg, then TBW $= 0.6 \times 50 = 30$ L.

$$\text{(TBW normal)} \times \text{(Na}^+ \text{ normal)} = \text{(TBW present)} \times \text{(Na}^+ \text{ present)}$$
$$X \times 140 = 30 \times 167 \qquad \text{(Eq. 3-5)}$$
$$\text{Deficit} = 35.7 - 30 = 5.7 \text{ L}$$

This calculated free-H_2O deficit exists at the time of presentation only. If loop diuretics are administered, then the Na concentration must be reassessed after the diuresis begins. Adequate free-H_2O repletion must occur simultaneously to prevent a further rise in the serum Na concentration.

CASE STUDY 3

Hypernatremia Secondary to Osmotic Diuresis

Mr. Tom Brown, a 60-year-old man with a 3-month history of urinary frequency, presented at the urology clinic complaining of decreasing urine output for one week. Upon physical examination the patient was alert and oriented, with a blood pressure of 170/95 mmHg, pulse of 96, respiration 22 bpm, and temperature of 99°F. His weight was 80 kg, and his chest was clear to P&A. Heart showed S_4 gallop, and abdomen a large, smooth, abdominal mass palpable to the umbilicus. The rectal exam revealed a large, firm prostate without nodules, and the extremities trace edema bilaterally.

LABORATORY DATA

Na 138 mEq/L	BUN 120 mg/dL
K 4.8 mEq/L	Creatinine 2.0 mg/dL
Cl 99 mEq/L	Glucose 100 mg/dL
HCO_3 24 mEq/L	

Urinalysis: negative for glucose, ketones, protein, blood
Microscopic exam: 3–5 WBC/HPF
Specific gravity: 1.008

He was admitted to the hospital with the presumptive diagnosis of bladder outlet obstruction secondary to prostatic hypertrophy. A foley catheter was inserted into his bladder. The patient was sedated because of anxiety. The following morning when he was seen on rounds, he was arousable but appeared disoriented. His blood pressure was 90/60, pulse was 110 when lying down; blood pressure was 80/50, pulse 130 when sitting up; respiratory rate was 15, and temperature was 99.2°F. The weight was not done, and the remainder of exam unchanged except he no longer had a palpable abdominal mass or edema

---

LABORATORY DATA

Na 158 mEq/L	BUN 60 mg/dL
K 3.2 mEq/L	Creatinine 1.6 mg/dL
Cl 124 mEq/L	Glucose 96 mg/dL
HCO_3 20 mEq/L	

Urine electrolytes: U_{Na} 80 mEq/L
I/O over the last 12 hours: intake 1000 ml/output (urine), 8.860 ml

---

Question 1. How do the history, physical exam, and laboratory data help in identifying the pathophysiologic mechanism responsible for the development of hypernatremia?

Question 2. How do his ECF and ICF compartments compare to those found in a normal individual?

Question 3. What other conditions are associated with hypertonic fluid losses?

Question 4. How would you manage his electrolyte and fluid balance?

---

1. **How do the history, physical exam, and laboratory data help in identifying the pathophysiologic mechanism responsible for the development of hypernatremia?**

History

The history is classic for bladder outlet obstruction, resulting from an enlarged prostate gland. The physical exam findings of a distended bladder, the large abdominal mass palpable to the umbilicus and a large firm prostate gland, confirms the diagnosis of bladder outlet obstruction. A markedly high BUN to creatinine ratio (60:1) is further confirmation of an obstructive uropathy. An ultrasound exam of the kidneys would most likely show bilateral hydronephrosis.

The placing of a foley catheter into the bladder allows the distended bladder to empty and relieves the bladder outlet obstruction. However, the diuresis which occurs is not limited to the urine retained in the bladder. Instead, a postobstructive diuresis often occurs because of 3 factors: (1) the high concentration of BUN that is filtered and excreted by the kidneys causes an *osmotic diuresis,* (2) the hydronephrotic kidney tubules are unable to reabsorb Na maximally, and (3) the hydronephrotic kidney tubules are resistant to ADH (causing NDI). All these factors result in the loss of large quantities of hypotonic urine (e.g., a urine having more H_2O than Na, but containing both). Generally, hypotonic urine has a UNa of 75–100 mEq/L. Following relief of the bladder outlet obstruction, the patient lost 8 liters of urine in 12 hours and (perhaps because of his sedation) only ingested one liter of H_2O.

Physical Exam

Assessing his volume status is particularly helpful in determining the cause of his hypernatremia. The physical exam indicates there is hypovolemia, and a reduced EABV, hypotension, tachycardia, and orthostatic hypotension without evidence of cardiac dysfunction. This presentation strongly suggests that the patient lost hypotonic fluids.

Laboratory Data

Hypernatremia (serum Na concentration of 158 mEq/L) as a result of losing both Na and H_2O, but more H_2O than Na. Note, the serum Na is not as high as that which occurs with free-H_2O loss (Case Study 1), but the patient is more symptomatic clinically because of the Na loss (i.e., hypotension).

Elevated Posm 316 + 5 + 20 = 314 mOsm/kg

Elevated effective Posm 316 + 5 = 321 mOsm/kg

Elevated BUN indicating prerenal azotemia

A high urine volume suggesting an osmotic diuresis is the etiology for the hypotonic fluid losses. Nonrenal causes of hypotonic fluid losses will result in a low volume of urine with a high specific gravity or high Uosm and a low UNa.

2. **How do his ECF and ICF compartments compare with those found in a normal individual (Fig. 3-2).**

Conditions causing a loss of hypotonic fluid are associated with a loss of a fluid that proportionally contains more H_2O than Na and by definition, has an osmolality less than plasma. To conceptualize hypotonic fluid, one can separate such fluids into a loss of free H_2O and a loss of isotonic solute. The calculation below may help to clarify this concept.

Example: Conceptualize the loss of 2 L of hypotonic fluid using ½ normal saline as an example (75 mEq Na + 75 mEq Cl for 150 mOsm). This fluid loss can be separated into

Loss of 1 L of normal saline		Loss of 1 L of free water
− 150 mEq	change in Na content	0
− 1000 mL	change in TBW	− 1000 mL
0	change in Posm	+ 2.5% (7.5 mOsm/l)
0	change in ICF volume	− 666 mL
− 1000 mL	change in ECF volume	− 333 mL
− 250 mL	change in plasma volume	− 83 mL

As the calculations show, the free water loss contracts both the ICF and ECF with two-thirds of the loss coming from the ICF and one-third of the loss from the ECF. However, loss of Na comes *only* from the ECF and in fact, for each one liter of normal saline (150 mEq Na; 150 mEq Cl) lost, 250 ml comes from the plasma (intravascular compartment). As Figure 3-7 indicates, loss of hypotonic fluids will cause significant ECF volume contraction. The consequence of ECF volume contraction is hypovolemia and the physical findings associated with that state: hypoten-

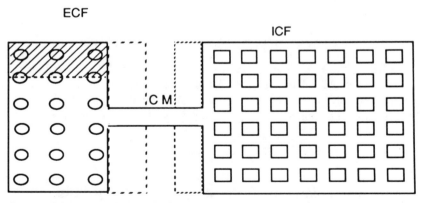

Fig. 3-7. Hypertonicity due to hypotonic fluid loss. Loss of hypotonic fluid from the ECF causes ECF and intravascular volume to contract to a greater degree than does the loss of pure H_2O. In this figure, it is assumed that the hypotonic fluid loss has an electrolyte content of about one-third of normal ECF. Although the total volume loss is only 50% more than with pure H_2O loss (compare Fig. 3-5), the concentration of the intravascular volume exceeds that of a pure H_2O loss by 150%. The degree of ICF contraction and the degree of hypertonicity are the same in the two cases. (CM, cell membranes.)

sion, tachycardia, orthostatic hypotension and other evidence for decreased effective circulating blood volume (increased BUN/creatinine ratio).

3. What other conditions are associated with hypotonic fluid losses?

There are either renal or nonrenal causes associated with hypotonic fluid losses.

Renal Causes
An osmotic diuresis will occur when large quantities of glucose, mannitol, glycerol or sorbitol, or BUN (e.g., associated with a postobstructive diuresis or high protein intake) are excreted in the urine. Each liter of urine will lose approximately 150 mEq of electrolytes in addition to the substance causing the diuresis.

Loop diuretics (e.g., furosemide) causes the loss of urine having 75 mEq Na and 75 mEq of an anion (one-half normal saline). If water is restricted, either orally or intravenously, hypernatremia will develop.

Nonrenal Causes
Certain gastrointestinal disorders are associated with the loss of large volumes of hypotonic fluids (e.g., osmotic diarrheas, fistulas, or diarrhea associated with lactulose).

4. How would you manage his electrolyte and fluid balance?

The first priority of treatment is correcting the Na loss, then correcting the water loss. Normal saline with 150 mEq Na and 150 mEq Cl is the fluid of choice, and it should be infused intravenously at a rapid rate until there is no further evidence of hypovolemia. This may require 1 to 2 L of normal saline over 30 to 90 minutes initially, followed by another 1 to 2 L infused more slowly using the blood pressure and pulse to assess adequate repletion. Since the concentration of Na in this solution is 150 mEq/L, if the patient's serum Na is greater than 150 mEq/L it will begin to fall slightly without administering any free-H_2O. Administering free H_2O to correct the hypernatremia should not be started until the patient is felt to be euvolemic.

The calculation of the free-H_2O deficit can be done using the same steps as in Case Study 1.

$$\text{Free-}H_2O \text{ deficit is} = 6.1 \text{ L } (48 - [(138/158)(48)]$$

Infusion of one-half of the H_2O deficit over the first 24 hours and the remainder over the next 24 to 48 hours is reasonable. This assumes that all ongoing urinary losses, Na, and H_2O losses are replaced immediately to prevent further hypotonic fluid losses. Measuring urinary lytes (UNa, UK) can help in determining the exact quantity of electrolyte replacement.

CASE STUDY 4

Hypernatremia Secondary to Hyperglycemia

Mr. Eli Jones, a 37-year-old hypertensive, obese male with a 3-day history of a cellulitis of his left leg, became progressively obtunded and was brought to the emergency room by his wife. On admission he responded to his name, but was disoriented, lethargic, and had a grand mal seizure. His blood pressure was 90/60; pulse was 100 and regular; and temperature was

100.2 rectally. His tissue turgor was decreased and he had no axillary sweat. He has no peripheral edema. No focal neurologic signs are present.

LABORATORY DATA

Na 135 mEq/L	BUN 30 mg/dL
K 35 mEq/L	Creatinine 1.6 mg/dL
Cl 100 mEq/L	Glucose 1800 mg/dL
HCO_3 24 mEq/L	

Urinalysis: dipstick − 4+ glucose; negative for ketones; sp. gravity 1.030; sediment: occasional WBC, no casts.
Weight (normal): 70 kg

Question 1. How do the history, physical exam, and laboratory data help in identifying the pathophysiologic mechanisms responsible for developing hypernatremia?

Question 2. What is his calculated Posm and plasma tonicity?

Question 3. How do his ECF and ICF compartments compare to those found in a normal individual?

Question 4. How would you explain a normal serum Na concentration in the presence of severe hyperglycemia?

Question 5. How do you determine the true serum Na concentration when hyperglycemia is present?

Question 6. How would you manage his electrolyte and fluid balance?

---

1. How do the history, physical exam, and laboratory data help in identifying the pathophysiologic mechanisms responsible for developing hypernatremia?

The history is consistent for hyperglycemia. The diagnosis becomes most likely if a history of polyuria and polydipsia can be elicited. The physical exam suggests both intravascular volume depletion or hypovolemia (hypotension, BP 90/60, and tachycardia, pulse of 100/min, and orthostatic hypotension) and cellular dehydration (mental status changes, i.e., brain cell dehydration, decreased tissue turgor, and decreased axillary sweat).

The laboratory data suggests the clinical condition hyperosmolar nonketotic coma (HNKC). This diagnosis is made when a serum glucose elevation (1800 mg/dL) is found without serum or urine ketones. Electrolytes indicate no acid-base disturbance. This diagnosis is distinguished from diabetic ketoacidosis (DKA), which is associated with ketonemia, ketonuria, and a serum acidemia (arterial blood Ph < 7.35). HNKC frequently occurs in either obese or elderly individuals without a previous history of diabetes mellitus who develop a condition often associated with insulin resistance, such as severe infections, pancreatitis, severe burns, stress of surgery, use of corticosteroids, and hyperalimentation fluids.

2. What is his calculated Posm and plasma tonicity?

$$\text{The Posm} = 2\ (135) + \frac{1800}{18} + \frac{30}{2.8} = 380\ \text{mOsm} \qquad \text{(Eq. 3-6)}$$

$$\text{Plasma Tonicity} = 2\ (135) + \frac{1800}{18} = 370\ \text{mOsm} \qquad \text{(Eq. 3-7)}$$

This individual is both *hyperosmolar* and *hypertonic*.

3. How do his ECF and ICF compartments compare with those found in a normal individual (Fig. 3-2)?

HNKC is associated with several pathophysiologic abnormalities that result in alterations to the ECF and ICF compartments.

Hyperglycemia
For every 100 mg/dL rise in the serum glucose concentration in the ECF, the Posm and effective Posm in the ECF rises approximately 5 mOsm (100 mg/dL/18 mg).

With a rise in the effective Posm, there is an initial shift of H_2O from the ICF to the ECF, dehydrating the ICF and expanding the ECF with H_2O (see Fig. 3-8A). As the diagram suggests, ECF expansion with H_2O dilutes the serum Na concentration, resulting in hyponatremia.

Osmotic Diuresis
Certain sugars that are freely filtered, but not reabsorbed, by the kidney tubules (e.g., mannitol, sorbitol, glycerol) or glucose or BUN that are freely filtered and not reabsorbed when their concentration exceeds the Tm for the kidney tubules will cause an osmotic diuresis. For each liter of urine lost, 1000 ml of H_2O will be lost, containing approximately 150 mOsm/L of the non-reabsorbed solute and 150 mOsm/L of electrolytes (generally a total of 150 mEq/L of Na or K and its anion, chloride, bicarbonate, sulphate, or phosphate). Since this urine contains only 150 mEq/L of electrolytes, it is hypotonic to serum, is classified as a loss of *hypotonic* fluid (see Fig. 3-4), and can be divided into loss of free H_2O and loss of Na.

Free-H_2O Loss. The excess glucose that is filtered by the kidney results in an osmotic diuresis. Twice as much H_2O as electrolytes is lost in every liter of urine. Large quantities of glucose excreted in the urine prevent the maximal reabsorption of water and cause an obligate water loss. Both the ECF and ICF compartments contract their volume but the ECF compartment contracts to normal. The ICF compartment contracts further since the ECF effective Posm rises with ECF contraction to normal (Fig. 3-8B).

Fig. 3-8. Hypertonicity and hypernatremia due to glucose addition (impermeant solute gain). **(A)** Glucose (solid circles) has been added to the ECF. Since glucose is relatively impermeant in the absence of insulin, it remains restricted to the ECF. The result is an increase in effective ECF solute concentration, expansion of the ECF, and contraction of the ICF (H_2O moves from ICF to ECF in response to the osmotic gradient). Note that the nonglucose solute content of the ECF (largely Na salts; open circles) remains the same, but the solute concentration decreases (producing hyponatremia). Thus, hyperglycemia can be associated with both hypertonicity and hyponatremia. **(B)** The alterations in the ECF and ICF as a result of osmotic diuresis with glucose are shown. The osmotic diuresis causes the loss of salt, glucose, and H_2O. The loss of Na salts (open circles) and glucose (closed circles) from the ECF results in contraction of that compartment. Since the ECF was initially expanded as a consequence of hyperglycemia, the osmotic diuresis returns the

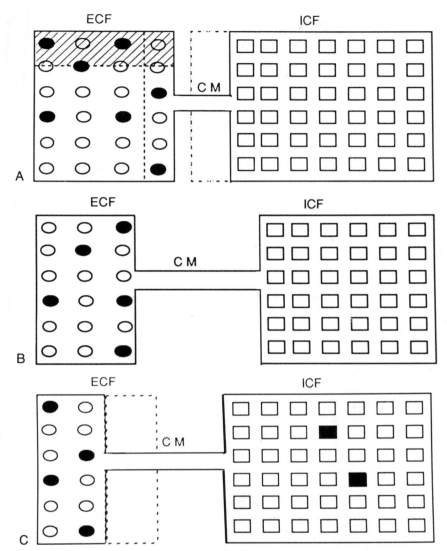

volume of this compartment toward normal; glucose (solid circles) contributes significantly to the overall concentration of impermeant ECF solutes. Water losses during the osmotic diuresis are derived from both the ICF (about two-thirds of the loss) and the ECF (about one-third of the loss). Therefore, the ICF, which was already contracted (in A), contracts further, but the ECR volume is maintained as a consequence of the ongoing hyperglycemia. (**C**) Alterations in ECF and ICF as a result of insulin administration. Insulin administration to treat hyperglycemia in Fig. B results in the movement of glucose from the ECF to the ICF; eventually, glucose is metabolized to CO_2 and H_2O in the ICF. The movement of glucose from the ECF to the ICF is associated with H_2O movement in the same direction as the osmolar gradient changes. As a result the ICF partially reexpands and ECF markedly contracts. The loss of glucose from the ECF, whether by osmotic diuresis or into the cells as a result of insulin administration, thus can produce profound EABV depletion and shock. Infusion of Na-containing solutions to maintain an adequate circulating volume is necessary prior to the administration of insulin when glucose is the predominant solute supporting the intravascular volume. (Modified from Feig PU, McCurdy DK: The hypertonic state. N Engl J Med 279: 1444, 1977.)

Sodium Loss. Each liter of urine lost as a result of the osmotic diuresis has 150 mEq of electrolytes, a significant portion being Na and its anion. Sodium is lost exclusively from the ECF compartment. Since the plasma compartment is one-fourth of the ECF compartment, 25% of all Na lost from the body will come from the plasma compartment. As Figure 3-8C indicates, loss of fluids containing significant quantities of Na causes marked contraction of the ECF compartment including the plasma compartment.

4. How would you explain a normal serum Na concentration in the presence of severe hyperglycemia?

This individual has lost significant quantities of both H_2O and Na as a result of an osmotic diuresis secondary to filtering large quantities of glucose. As Figure 3-8 indicates, the initial expansion of the ECF from hyperglycemia (which is associated with hyponatremia), converts to contraction of the ECF and ICF with the loss of salt and H_2O from the osmotic diuresis. As the ECF contracts, the serum Na concentration rises.

5. How do you determine the true serum Na concentration when hyperglycemia is present?

The true Na or corrected Na concentration is the serum Na concentration that would be expected if the glucose concentration could be normalized immediately (e.g., 100 mg/dL).

The correction factor assumes that the serum sodium concentration will rise 1.6 mEq/L for each 100 mg/dL drop in glucose concentration.

In this case, one would multiply 17×1.6 mEq/L (glucose is elevated 1700 mg above normal). A total of 27 mEq/L would be added to the serum Na concentration that existed when the glucose concentration was 1800 mg/dL. The true Na or corrected Na is $135 + 27 = 162$ mEq/L. This value is a good measure of the quantity of free H_2O lost as a consequence of the osmotic diuresis. Since the true serum Na concentration indicates hypernatremia, this individual has lost significant quantities of free H_2O.

6. How would you manage his electrolyte and fluid balance?

Correct the Na Deficit
The first priority of therapy is to replace NaCl losses with intravenous normal saline solutions. In this individual, with physical exam findings indicative of hypovolemia and an elevated true serum Na concentration indicative of an osmotic diuresis, the repletion of his ECF compartment with saline is of prime importance. Infusion of 2 or 3 liters of normal saline over 1 to 2 hours may be necessary to sufficiently expand the ECF compartment *before* treating his hyperglycemia. It is important to remember that his elevated glucose concentration is contributing significantly to his Posm and effective Posm. Giving insulin, which will cause glucose to move intercellularly *before* there is adequate sodium replacement to maintain the ECF compartment volume, will cause further contraction of the ECF compartment, which clinically would result in the development of shock.

Correction of the H_2O Deficit
The free-H_2O deficit can be calculated using the true or corrected serum sodium concentration. In this individual, his present serum sodium concentration is 162 mEq/L when his serum glucose concentration is 1800 mg/dL. At that point in time, his free H_2O deficit is 5.7 L: $42 - [(140 \times 42)/162]$.

Replacement of free H_2O should be done *slowly*. No more than half of the replacement should occur in the first 24 hours, with the remainder occurring over the next 24 to 48 hours. This can be accomplished with D 5/w once the serum glucose concentration is below 300 mg/dL or with 25% normal saline if glucose-free solutions are needed. The presence of idiogenic osmoles in brain cells makes cerebral edema a real possibility if correction of the H_2O deficit is too rapid.

Insulin Replacement

Individuals with HNKC may resolve their hyperglycemia with replacement of their fluid losses and treatment of their underlying medical condition (e.g., infection). However, with significantly elevated concentrations of glucose (>500 mg/dL), standard medical treatment consists of a continuous infusion of small doses of insulin (2–5 units/h), which should lower the glucose concentration slowly.

Potassium Replacement

Individuals with HNKC may have total body K depletion since one of the electrolytes lost in an osmotic diuresis is K. Treating the hyperglycemia with insulin will shift K intracellularly, and further lower serum K. Therefore, K supplements (KCl) are usually necessary for most individuals and are added as necessary to intravenous solutions after assuring that the individual has an adequate urine output. The maximum safe infusion rate for KCl is 40 mEq/h.

4

Potassium Homeostasis

Kumar Sharma
Malcolm Cox

Hospitalized patients will have their plasma potassium concentration (pK) checked many times during a typical stay. This is the case for many outpatients as well. Why do physicians pay so much attention to the pK? The major reason is that both *hypokalemia* and *hyperkalemia* can cause life-threatening arrhythmias. In addition, because pK is affected by so many different factors, abnormalities in pK are among the more common electrolyte disturbances encountered in clinical medicine.

Total body K (TBK) approximates 60 mEq/kg in a 20-year-old lean male, of which 90% is intracellular (mainly in muscle) and only 2% is extracellular; the bulk of the remainder is inaccessible in bone.

The intracellular to extracellular K concentration ratio determines the cell membrane potential, and so K has a central role in determining the cell membrane potential. The Na^+,K^+-ATPase pump is responsible for maintaining the intracellular K concentration (150 mEq/L) greater than the extracellular fluid K concentration (4.5 mEq/L). Potassium diffuses out of the cell through specific channels in the cell membrane, but at the same time intracellular anions (largely proteins and organic phosphates) are excluded from following K out of the cell. The cell membrane is relatively impermeable to Na (as compared to K), so Na is largely restricted to the extracellular fluid. The Na that does "leak" into the cell is extruded by the Na^+,K^+-ATPase.

The resting membrane potential (Em) of the cell can be derived from the Goldman-Hodgkin-Katz constant field equation:

$$Em = -61 \log \frac{r(K^+)ICF + 0.01(Na^+)ICF}{r(K^+)ECF + 0.01(Na^+)ECF} = -86 \text{ mv} \qquad \text{(Eq. 4-1)}$$

where r is the 3:2 transport ratio of the electrogenic Na pump (Na^+,K^+-ATPase) and 0.01 is the membrane permeability of Na relative to that of K. Thus, Em is largely dependent on the intracellular to extracellular K ratio, small changes in which have dramatic effects on Em. As

71

the ratio (K)ICF/(K)ECF increases, the cell hyperpolarizes (becomes more negative). As the ratio falls, the cell depolarizes (becomes less negative). Both of these situations impair action potential generation and the functioning of cardiac and skeletal muscle.

Given its importance in determining the cell membrane potential, it is not surprising that pK is tightly regulated. Two separate but cooperative systems maintain K homeostasis, regulating the distribution of K across cell membranes (internal K balance) and total body K content (external K balance) (Fig. 4-1).

INTERNAL POTASSIUM BALANCE

Relatively small changes in internal K balance can have profound sequelae. Given that the normal extracellular fluid K content is only about 70 mEq, pK would double if as little as 2% of intracellular K were to translocate into the extracellular fluid. Similarly, if the volume of distribution of K was restricted to the extracellular fluid, lethal hyperkalemia would follow a large meal. Were it not for redistribution of K, the loss of only 70 mEq of K in the stool or urine would, if unreplaced, lead to lethal hypokalemia. Thus, adjustments in internal K balance are critical features of the defense against both hyperkalemia and hypokalemia.

Regulation by Hormones

Internal K balance is regulated by hormones. *Insulin* is the most important hormonal regulator of internal K balance (Fig. 4-2). Basal circulating insulin levels are a prerequisite for normal distribution of K across cell membranes. Insulin promotes K uptake by muscle, liver, and adipose

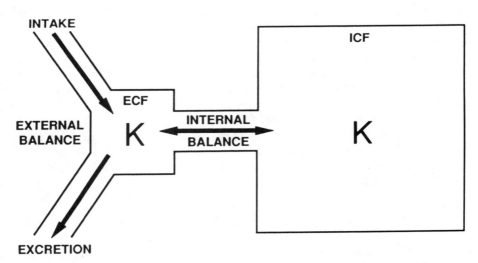

Fig. 4-1. Internal and external potassium balance (ECF and ICF, extracellular and intracellular fluid, respectively).

INSULIN
β-ADRENERGIC AGONISTS
ALDOSTERONE
METABOLIC ALKALOSIS

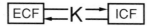

INORGANIC ACIDOSIS
α-ADRENERGIC AGONISTS
β-ADRENERGIC ANTAGONISTS
HYPERTONICITY

Fig. 4-2. Factors affecting internal potassium balance (ECF and ICF, extracellular and intracellular fluid, respectively).

tissue. The clinical importance of insulin in K homeostasis is best exemplified by the reduction in K tolerance that characterizes diabetes mellitus.

Although K is a potent insulin secretogogue, the degree of hyperkalemia required to stimulate pancreatic insulin release appears to be at the higher end of the physiologic range. Thus, while changes in circulating insulin levels may be important in the defense against severe hyperkalemia, it is uncertain whether K-stimulated insulin release forms part of this physiologic feedback loop during more modest increments in pK.

Catecholamines also have important effects on internal K balance: β-adrenergic receptor activation increases cellular K uptake and α-adrenergic receptor activation decreases cellular uptake and promotes hepatic K release. Thus, epinephrine (a combined α- and β-agonist) causes a transient increase in pK followed by a more sustained decrease. Likewise, β-receptor blockade impairs K tolerance.

Whether *aldosterone* has direct effects on internal K balance has been controversial for many years. However, recent studies have shown that mineralocorticoids do enhance cellular K uptake. Because physiological increases in pK also stimulate aldosterone secretion, aldosterone may have a role in regulating internal K balance—participating, with insulin, in the defense against hyperkalemia.

Acid-Base Balance

Although the underlying cellular mechanisms are still poorly understood, our understanding of the effects of acid-base disturbances on internal K balance has undergone considerable revision in recent years. The long held dogma that changes in pK are always inversely proportional to changes in extracellular fluid pH is now recognized as a simplistic overgeneralization. Rather, the effects of acid-base disturbances on K distribution depend on both the specific nature and the duration of the disturbance. Concurrent effects of acid-base balance on renal K excretion also influence the relationship between pH and pK, as do a variety of coincidental factors, such as renal function, the prevailing hormonal milieu, and body fluid tonicity. Thus, the effect of a particular acid-base disturbance on pK is not always readily predictable.

The most consistent relationship between changes in pH and pK occurs in *acute inorganic acidosis*, pK increasing by about 0.8 mEq/L for each 0.1 unit decline in extracellular fluid pH. In contrast, provided that renal K excretory capacity is intact, *chronic inorganic acidoses* are generally accompanied by hypokalemia (rather than hyperkalemia) because of the kaliuresis that typically accompanies the transition from the acute acid-base disturbance to the chronic steady state. Thus, hypokalemia is an essential element of both proximal and classic distal renal tubular acidosis.

Unlike inorganic acidoses, *organic acidoses* do not affect K distribution. Thus, neither uncomplicated lactic acidosis nor alcoholic ketoacidosis are associated with hyperkalemia. However, factors occurring coincident with the acidosis, either by affecting K distribution or by altering renal K handling, may alter pK.

Under most circumstances *acute metabolic alkalosis,* as seen with intravenous $NaHCO_3$ administration, results in only a modest fall in pK (0.3 mEq/L for every 0.1 unit rise in extracellular fluid pH). *Chronic metabolic alkalosis,* as seen with prolonged vomiting or nasogastric suction, is almost invariably associated with hypokalemia. However, the hypokalemia in this instance primarily results from the accompanying kaliuresis and is usually associated with profound K depletion.

Unlike metabolic disorders, respiratory disorders are not usually associated with clinically significant alterations in pK.

Body Fluid Tonicity

Hypertonicity shifts K out of cells, possibly because the associated cell shrinkage increases the intracellular to extracellular fluid K gradient. However, whether hyperkalemia actually occurs depends on the integrity of the overall K homeostatic system. Glucose-induced hyperkalemia is the most clinically important example of this phenomenon, occurring in individuals with insulin and/or mineralocorticoid deficiency. *Hypotonicity* does not appear to affect K distribution.

TOTAL BODY POTASSIUM CONTENT

Total body K (TBK) content is determined by external K balance, i.e., by the difference between K intake and K excretion. While moment to moment correlations between pK and TBK are imperfect because of transitory changes in internal K balance, sustained perturbations in pK generally imply disorders of external balance, that is, they are associated with alterations in TBK.

A typical American ingests 50 to 150 mEq K daily. Normally, only about 10 to 20 mEq of dietary K is excreted in the stool but the gastrointestinal tract may account for a greater proportion of total K elimination in patients with renal insufficiency or diarrhea. Sweat has a mean K concentration of only about 10 mEq/L and the skin is generally not an important source of loss.

TBK stores are held constant by varying urinary K excretion to match K intake. Under normal circumstances, 90% of dietary K is excreted in the urine and the kidney can vary the amount excreted from as little as 5 to 10 to as much as 700 to 1000 mEq daily. The kidney is particularly well adapted to accommodate chronic increases in K intake, quantitatively excreting the new dietary load within a few days. The kidney is only able to excrete part of an acute K load, however, and the remainder is translocated into the cells. This dual defense against hyperkalemia can be easily overwhelmed by overly aggressive K replacement therapy, especially if renal K excretion or cellular K uptake is impaired. The kidney is also able to accommodate decreases in K intake, but it takes a week or more before renal K conservation becomes maximal. It is

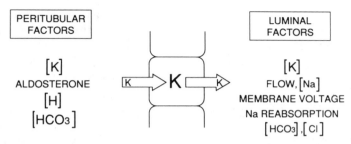

Fig. 4-3. Factors affecting renal potassium secretion. ([K], [H], [HCO$_3$], [Na], [Cl] = Potassium, proton, bicarbonate, sodium, and chloride concentrations, respectively).

unusual for insufficient intake to be the sole cause of K depletion; however, inadequate intake may contribute whenever urinary or gastrointestinal K excretion is excessive.

URINARY POTASSIUM EXCRETION

Potassium is freely filtered by the glomerulus. Nearly all the filtered K is reabsorbed in the proximal tubule and the ascending limb of Henle's loop. Most excreted K is derived from K secretion in more distal portions of the nephron (distal convoluted tubule, connecting tubule, and cortical collecting duct). Urinary K excretion is largely regulated by appropriate alterations in the magnitude of distal tubular K secretion (Fig. 4-3). Increases in K intake or hyperkalemia enhance distal tubular K secretion while hypokalemia or K depletion are associated with reductions in K secretion. Thus, the renal adaptation to alterations in K balance is mediated by adjustments in distal tubular K secretion. Aldosterone is the major hormonal regulator of distal tubular K secretion. Sodium balance and acid-base balance also modulate urinary K excretion, in large part by altering distal K secretion.

Aldosterone

Hyperkalemia enhances aldosterone secretion, so in many situations in which K intake and excretion are elevated, pK and circulating aldosterone levels both rise. While changes in either variable alone are sufficient to enhance K secretion, under normal circumstances pK (and/or TBK) and aldosterone act cooperatively to set the precise K secretory rate. Given the importance of aldosterone in regulating external K balance, it is not surprising that hyperkalemia is a common manifestation of hypoaldosteronism and pseudohypoaldosteronism (renal unresponsiveness to aldosterone) and that hypokalemia and K depletion are prominent features of hyperaldosteronism.

Sodium Balance and Tubular Flow

Urinary Na and K excretion generally change in parallel. For example, increasing Na excretion (e.g., volume expansion, osmotic diuresis, diuretic administration) enhances K excretion—both from inhibition of proximal tubular and ascending limb of Henle K reabsorption and from enhanced distal tubular K secretion. Distal Na delivery is the product of distal tubular fluid Na concentration and flow. However, because the distal tubular fluid Na concentration rarely falls to levels that limit K secretion, increased flow may be the dominant factor linking kaliuresis and natriuresis. Distal tubular K secretion varies directly with luminal flow because removal of secreted K maintains the electrochemical gradient for continued movement of K from cell to lumen.

Acid-Base Balance

A complete understanding of the interrelationships between acid-base balance and urinary K excretion has yet to be achieved. However, it is clear that the effects of acid-base disturbances on distal tubular K secretion depend on both the nature and duration of the disturbance. Thus, *acute alkalosis* stimulates, and *acute acidosis* inhibits, distal tubular K secretion. *Chronic metabolic alkalosis* is almost invariably associated with severe K depletion, the accelerated K secretory rate that accompanies the onset of the disturbance persisting throughout the transition to the new steady state. Interestingly, *chronic metabolic acidosis* is also associated with K depletion, the transition from acute to chronic metabolic acidosis being associated with increased (rather than decreased) K secretion.

Flow-related enhancement of distal K secretion undoubtedly contributes to the K depletion observed in both of these chronic acid-base disorders, the kaliuresis generally being accompanied by natriuresis (NaCl in the case of metabolic acidosis and $NaHCO_3$ in the case of metabolic alkalosis). In chronic metabolic alkalosis, however, factors other than increased flow are also important. The increased plasma HCO_3/Cl ratio so characteristic of this disorder, when translated to the luminal environment of the distal tubule, enhances K secretion. Replacement of the more permeable Cl with the relatively less permeable HCO_3 increases transepithelial potential difference (lumen negative), thereby increasing K secretion. A very low luminal Cl concentration, in and of itself, may also enhance K secretion.

Respiratory disorders are usually not associated with clinically significant alterations in external K balance.

GENERAL READINGS

Bia MJ, DeFronzo RA: Extrarenal potassium homeostasis. Am J Physiol 240:F257, 1981

Field MJ, Giebisch GJ: Hormonal control of renal potassium excretion. Kidney Int 276:379, 1985

Ponce SP, Jennings AE, Madias NE, Harrington JT: Drug-induced hyperkalemia. Medicine 64:357, 1985

Rose BD: Clinical Physiology of Acid-Base and Electrolyte Disorders. 3rd Ed., McGraw-Hill, New York, 1989

Sebastian A, Schambelan M: Renal hyperkalemia. Sem Nephrol 7:223, 1987

Smith JD, Bia MJ, DeFronzo RA: Clinical disorders of potassium metabolism. p. 413. In Arieff AI, DeFronzo RA (eds): Fluid, Electrolyte and Acid-Base Disorders. Churchill Livingstone, New York, 1985

Sterns RH, Cox M, Feig PU, Singer I: Internal potassium balance and the control of the plasma potassium concentration. Medicine 60:339, 1981

Sterns RH, Spital A: Disorders of internal potassium balance. Sem Nephrol 7:206, 1987

Tannen RL: Potassium Disorders. p. 195. In Kokko JH, Tanner RL (eds): Fluids and Electrolytes. 2nd Ed., WB Saunders Co., Philadelphia, 1990

Weisberg LS, Szerlip HM, Cox M: Disorders of potassium homeostasis in critically ill patients. Critical Care Clinics 5:835, 1987

Wright FS: Renal potassium handling. Sem Nephrol 7:174, 1987

Young D: Analysis of long-term potassium regulation. Endocrine Rev 6:24, 1985

CASE STUDY 1

An Isolated Lab Value of Hyperkalemia

A 25-year-old healthy male, Mr. Norm Testa, underwent baseline blood tests before being accepted as a volunteer in a clinical study. Repeated blood samples revealed K levels between 5.8 and 6.2 mEq/L.

LABORATORY DATA

K 5.8–6.2 mEq/L   EKG normal

Question 1. Does this situation warrant a full evaluation for hyperkalemia?
Question 2. How should the blood for measuring K levels be obtained?

---

1. Does this situation warrant a full evaluation for hyperkalemia?

Whenever an unexpected abnormal test is obtained, consider the possibility of a spurious result before initiating an exhaustive search for nonexistent disorders. In obtaining blood samples patients are often asked to make a fist prior to the sample being withdrawn. Repeated vigorous fist clenching releases K into the extracellular fluid, resulting in *local venous hyperkalemia*—hyperkalemia that is not present outside the venous circulation of the limb being sampled.[1]

Another cause of spurious hyperkalemia is in vitro cell lysis occurring in the blood collection tube as K-rich protoplasm is released into the fluid phase. The most common cause of so-called *pseudohyperkalemia* is hemolysis,[2] which can usually be detected by visual inspection, since the serum contains free hemoglobin. Other causes of pseudohyperkalemia include lysis of platelets or white blood cells in settings of marked thrombocytosis[3] or leukocytosis.[4] In rare instances, pseudohyperkalemia has been associated with mononucleosis[5] or familial disorders.[6]

Pseudohyperkalemia is generally only seen when serum, rather than plasma, is used for the measurement of blood K levels. Provided that cells are rapidly separated from plasma, the plasma K concentration generally provides an accurate assessment of the true extracellular fluid K concentration. However, when white blood cells are left in prolonged contact with plasma at 4°C they lose K and pseudohyperkalemia can occur.[4] Interestingly, extreme leukocytosis has been associated with pseudo*hypo*kalemia as well. If white blood cells are left in contact with plasma for extended periods at room temperature they continue to be metabolically active, taking up K in the process.[7]

2. How should the blood for measuring K levels be obtained?

Blood should be collected carefully and processed promptly. A free-flowing venous specimen is best. If a tourniquet is used it should only be employed briefly and the fist should not be repeatedly clenched. To decrease the risk of hemolysis, medium caliber needles should be employed and excessive negative pressure avoided. A heparinized specimen (plasma) is best, especially in patients with marked thrombocytosis or leukocytosis. Samples should remain at room temperature and plasma should be separated from cells within an hour of venipuncture.

If, after obtaining the specimen correctly, the hyperkalemia is verified, a complete evaluation is warranted. Such a work up would be designed to identify disturbances in both internal and external K homeostasis.

CASE STUDY 2

Hyperkalemia Secondary to Exogenous Intake

A 40-year-old depressed male, Mr. Bill Popper, ingested 75 Micro-K tablets in a suicide attempt. He was brought to the emergency room about 5 hours later complaining of diffuse weakness.

LABORATORY DATA

K 7.0 mEq/L   EKG widened QRS complex, peaked T waves

Question 1. What is the cause of the hyperkalemia?
Question 2. Why does the patient have muscle weakness?
Question 3. What are the EKG manifestations of hyperkalemia?
Question 4. What therapies are available for the emergency treatment of severe hyperkalemia?

---

1. What is the cause of the hyperkalemia?

The cause of the hyperkalemia is obvious—the ingestion of large amounts of K over a very short period of time. Each 600 mg tablet of Micro-K contains 8 mEq of K, so 75 tablets provide 600 mEq. Assuming normal renal function, approximately 50% (300 mEq) would be excreted in the urine over 3 hours and two-thirds to three-quarters of the remainder would be translocated intracellularly.[8] This would leave 75 to 100 mEq in the extracellular fluid, easily explaining the near doubling of the blood K concentration.

2. Why does the patient have muscle weakness?

The muscle weakness results from a decrease in the resting membrane potential (cell depolarization).[9] As the resting potential approaches the threshold potential, excitable cells are unable to sustain action potentials, causing weakness and paralysis.

3. What are the EKG manifestations of hyperkalemia?

The EKG findings of hyperkalemia are due to abnormal cardiac muscle depolarization and repolarization.[10] The initial effect of hyperkalemia is to produce narrow, peaked T waves and a shortened QT interval. With increasing severity, the QRS complex widens and the P wave disappears. Prior to ventricular asystole or fibrillation, a sine wave pattern is typically seen as the widened QRS complex merges with the T wave.

Although these EKG manifestations correlate with the magnitude of the hyperkalemia, the association is quite variable. For example, normal T waves do not exclude hyperkalemia.[11] Unless extreme, it is also difficult to know whether T wave "peaking" is present or not. The only truly reliable way to ascertain this is by comparison to a cardiogram taken during normokalemia. Because the progression from milder to more severe manifestations is unpredictable and because ventricular asystole or fibrillation may suddenly supervene, patients with more than mild T wave abnormalities should be treated promptly. So should patients with pK greater than 6.0 mEq/L, even if there are no EKG changes.

4. What therapies are available for the emergency treatment of severe hypokalemia?

The available therapies for life-threatening hyperkalemia can be grouped into three categories: *antagonism, redistribution,* and *elimination.* In a patient such as the one described, the first priority is to reduce cardiac irritability. By decreasing the threshold potential (making it less negative, thereby moving it further from the resting potential), calcium protects against the depolarizing effects of hyperkalemia.[10,12] Conversely, hypocalcemia predisposes to the cardiotoxicity of hyperkalemia by increasing the threshold potential (thereby moving it closer to the resting potential).[13] Calcium antagonism is rapid: the onset of action is only a few minutes.

Calcium is usually administered as a 10% calcium gluconate solution by slow IV push (10 mL of a 10% solution contains 93 mg Ca and should be infused over 1 to 5 minutes with continuous EKG monitoring). This can be repeated if the EKG changes do not resolve within 5 minutes. Whether to employ Ca depends on the severity of the EKG changes—the absence of P waves and QRS widening indicate serious toxicity and the possibility of imminent ventricular asystole or fibrillation. T wave peaking is not, by itself, an indication for Ca treatment. Ca should not be employed to treat hyperkalemia in patients with digitalis intoxication.[14]

The fact that insulin redistributes K into cells[15,16] can be used to therapeutic advantage in patients with life-threatening hyperkalemia. The intravenous administration of 25 to 50 g glucose (as 5% or 10% dextrose-in-water) will stimulate endogenous insulin secretion in non-diabetic patients and lower pK by 1 to 2 mEq/L within 30 to 60 minutes; the effect usually lasts for several hours. The concomitant administration of 10 to 20 units of regular insulin serves to maximize cellular K uptake and is mandatory in diabetic patients. Complications include hypoglycemia and hyperglycemia. Severe hyperglycemia can promote hyperkalemia[17] and should be avoided.

The administration of sodium bicarbonate (usually 45 to 90 mEq IV over 15 to 30 minutes) also results in cellular K uptake; this effect may be independent of changes in pH, correlating rather with the increase in the serum HCO_3 concentration.[18] The plasma K concentration begins to fall within 5 to 10 minutes and may persist for an hour or two. Interestingly, HCO_3 may be more effective in lowering pK in hyperkalemic than in normokalemic individuals.[19] In contrast to its efficacy in patients with normal renal function or only modest renal insufficiency, HCO_3 has been reported to be ineffective in patients on maintenance hemodialysis.[20] Until additional studies are performed, it would seem prudent not to rely on HCO_3 as the sole agent for the emergency treatment of hyperkalemia in the end-stage renal disease population. Complications of bicarbonate therapy include volume overload and metabolic alkalosis. Bicarbonate can be administered along with glucose and insulin. Calcium should never be added to bicarbonate-containing solutions because of the risk of precipitation of insoluble calcium salts.

Beta-adrenergic agonists also promote cellular K uptake[21] and have been used to reverse hyperkalemia.[22] Unfortunately, the response is variable and β-agonists are not presently recommended for the general treatment of hyperkalemia. Because they can be administered as inhalants, however, they may be of benefit in patients without immediate IV access. They have also been used successfully in the prophylaxis of hyperkalemic periodic paralysis.[23]

The redistribution of K into cells decreases the risk of cardiac toxicity, but the excess K still must be removed from the body. "Elimination" can be accomplished with cation exchange resins, diuretics or dialysis. Sodium polystyrene sulfonate (Kayexalate) is the most widely used resin, exchanging Na for K in the gut and removing K in the stool.[24] Each gram of resin binds 1 mEq K and releases 1 to 2 mEq of Na.

Kayexalate (25–50 g) is usually given orally together with 15 to 30 mL of 70% sorbitol to act as a cathartic, the mixture being diluted with H_2O as necessary. Kayexalate can also be given as a retention enema in patients who cannot take it by mouth. In this case, 50 to 100 grams of resin in 100 to 200 ml H_2O are inserted into the rectum with a foley catheter and retained for at least 60 minutes. Because other cations also bind to the resin, antacids containing magnesium, calcium, or aluminum should be withheld. The major side effects of Kayexalate are gastrointestinal intolerance, often including severe diarrhea, and Na overload. Kayexalate should not be used in patients with ileus or bowel obstruction.

Loop diuretics can be used to enhance K secretion by enhancing distal flow,[25] but they are rarely helpful in management of acute, severe hyperkalemia. Dialysis is available for patients with renal insufficiency; hemodialysis is the preferred modality in emergency situations.[26]

CASE STUDY 3

Hyperkalemia Associated with Diabetes Mellitus

Mr. Bob Sulen, a 20-year-old male with insulin-dependent diabetes mellitus of 4 years duration, was admitted after running out of insulin 3 days ago. His only complaints are polyuria and polydipsia. Physical exam is remarkable for mild orthostatic tachycardia and hypotension, a respiratory rate of 26/min, and the fruity odor of his breath.

LABORATORY DATA

Na 130 mEq/L	BUN 35 mg/dL
Cl 100 mEq/L	Creatinine 1.5 mg/dL
K 6.2 mEq/L	Glucose 670 mg/dL
HCO_3 10 mEq/L	

Urinalysis: 4+ glucose, 4+ ketones and trace protein
Arterial blood gas: pH 7.20, pCO_2 21, pO_2 105 and HCO_3 8
EKG shows peaked T waves

Question 1. What are the potential causes of hyperkalemia in this patient, and which do you think best explain it?
Question 2. What is the patient's total body K likely to be: high, normal or low?
Question 3. What are the implications for therapy?

---

1. **What are the potential causes of hyperkalemia in this patient, and which do you think best explain it?**

Changes in internal K balance that might be considered are *insulin deficiency, hyperglycemia,* and *acidemia.* The patient is an insulin-dependent diabetic who has not taken insulin for 3 days, so there is little question that he is insulin deficient. The hyperglycemia and anion gap metabolic acidosis (almost certainly ketoacidosis given the history and positive urinary ketones) bear further testament to insulin deficiency. The hypoinsulism[27] and hyperglycemia[17] lead to a net shift of K out of cells and can more than adequately explain the hyperkalemia.

Because acid-base disorders are known to influence internal K balance,[28,29] it is also reasonable to question whether acidemia has a role in the hyperkalemia in this patient. Depending on the nature of the conjugate base (anion), all acids can be categorized into inorganic (mineral) or organic acids. Hydrochloric acid (Cl^-), phosphoric acid ($H_3PO_4{}^-/H_2PO_4{}^=$) and sulfuric acid ($SO_4{}^=$) are inorganic acids (and their conjugate bases) that accumulate in patients with renal tubular acidosis or renal insufficiency. Acetoacetic acid (acetoacetate$^-$), β-hydroxybutyric acid (β-hydroxybutyrate$^-$) and lactic acid (lactate$^-$) are examples of organic acids (and their conjugate bases).

These distinctions are important because inorganic and organic acidoses have distinctly different effects on internal K balance.[30] Although inorganic acidosis is associated with a net redistribution of K out of cells (and can, therefore, cause hyperkalemia), organic acidosis, even when severe, is not. A complete explanation of the different behavior of inorganic and organic acids has proven elusive. However, differences in the volume of distribution of inorganic versus organic anions are likely to be important.[30] For example, Cl^- is effectively excluded from the intracellular fluid by a very low cell membrane permeability, whereas organic anions, in their undissociated form, penetrate cells quite readily. In order to maintain electroneutrality, intracellular buffering of an inorganic acid necessitates the efflux of cellular cations, predominantly K—hence the penchant for hyperkalemia with inorganic acidosis. Such is not the case with organic acidoses because entry of the undissociated acid into the cell does not disturb electroneutrality. Whatever the underlying cellular mechanisms, however, it is clear from both experimental[30] and clinical[31,32] studies that organic acidoses are not associated with hyperkalemia. Thus, this patient's hyperkalemia cannot be ascribed to the diabetic ketoacidosis.

Changes in external balance that might be considered in this patient revolve around decreased renal K excretion: *renal insufficiency, hypoaldosteronism,* and *decreased distal flow.* The mild prerenal azotemia (elevated BUN/Creatinine ratio) is likely the result of volume depletion secondary to the osmotic diuresis (glycosuria, ketonuria), rather than being due to intrinsic renal disease. In any event, renal K excretion is generally well preserved in patients with renal insufficiency until GFR falls below 10% of normal,[33] which is clearly not the case here. It is also worth mentioning that ketonemia falsely elevates the serum Creatinine concentration.[34]

Diabetics have a high incidence of *hyporeninemic hypoaldosteronism,*[35] which would limit distal tubular K secretory ability. From the information provided it is impossible to assess this possibility. However, the patient's aldosterone secretory ability could be formally evaluated (see Case Study 4) if hyperkalemia continues despite correction of the hypoinsulism and hyperglycemia.

While decreased distal flow certainly limits K secretory capacity, such is not the case here. Although the patient is volume depleted (orthostatic hypotension, prerenal azotemia), this is the consequence of an ongoing osmotic diuresis (glycosuria, ketonuria) and he has been polyuric, rather than oliguric, over the past several days.

2. What is the patient's total body K likely to be: high, low, or normal?

Osmotic diureses are characterized by large urinary losses of Na, K, and H_2O.[36] Solute and water reabsorption in the proximal tubule and loop of Henle are decreased, fluid delivery to the distal nephron is increased, and renal K secretion is enhanced.[37] Secondary hyperaldosteronism and increased delivery of relatively nonreabsorbable ketone anions may also contribute to the enhanced K secretion.[37] Thus, this patient is likely to have suffered large urinary K losses over the course of the illness. It is by no means unusual for uncontrolled diabetics to be markedly K depleted (osmotic diuresis) despite hyperkalemia (insulin deficiency, hypertonicity).[37,38]

3. What are the implications for therapy?

This has important implications for therapy. As soon as insulin is administered and K is translocated into cells, the hyperkalemia will be replaced by hypokalemia.[39] This is a common and dangerous (cardiac arrhythmias) sequence of events in the treatment of diabetic ketoacidosis unless forstalled by the early institution of K replacement therapy.

CASE STUDY 4

Hyperkalemia Associated with Mild Renal Insufficiency

Mr. Ed Ace, a 61-year-old obese male with a 14-year history of noninsulin-dependent diabetes mellitus, was admitted to the hospital with chest pain. His only medication is glypizide 5 mg/d. The blood pressure was 180/100 mmHg supine, the lungs were clear and trace pretibial edema was present. He was placed on a low Na diet and fluid restriction and started on nitrates and captopril 25 mg bid. Cardiac enzymes rule out a myocardial infarction. A repeat chemistry profile was obtained on the third hospital day, at which time his blood pressure was 150/90 mmHg supine and 138/85 mmHg erect, the lungs were clear and the edema had resolved.

LABORATORY DATA

Admission

Na 138 mEq/L	HCO_3 18 Eq/L	Creatinine 1.9 mg/dL
Cl 110 mEq/L	BUN 27 mg/dL	Glucose 260 mg/dL
K 5 mEq/L		

Urinalysis: 3+ protein, trace ketones, pH 5.5

Day 3

Na 136 mEq/L	HCO_3 15 mEq/L	Creatinine 2.0 mg/dL
Cl 115 mEq/L	BUN 35 mg/dL	Glucose 195 mg/dL
K 5.8 mEq/L		

An EKG shows no signs of hyperkalemia.
ABG: pH 7.31, pCO_2 30, pO_2 89, HCO_3 14

Question 1. What are the potential causes of hyperkalemia in this patient?
Question 2. Which of these causes best explains this patient's current problem?
Question 3. How would you substantiate the diagnosis?
Question 4. How would you treat the hyperkalemia?

===

1. What are the potential causes of hyperkalemia in this patient?

The patient has longstanding adult-onset diabetes mellitus and mild renal insufficiency. The plasma K concentration was normal on admission and rose in association with a fall in the blood HCO_3 level. Review of the diet showed that the patient was compliant with his low (60 mEq) Na diet and that he had a fluid intake of about 1200 ml per day. *Dietary K intake* was estimated to be about 80 mEq/day. He was not receiving *K supplements*,[40] *K-containing drugs* (such as K salts of penicillin antibiotics),[41] or *salt substitutes* (which are low in Na but high in K).[42] Repeated questioning also ascertained that family and visitors were not bringing him fruit juices or fresh or dried fruit, all of which contain large amounts of K.[43] Thus, the patient's K intake did not

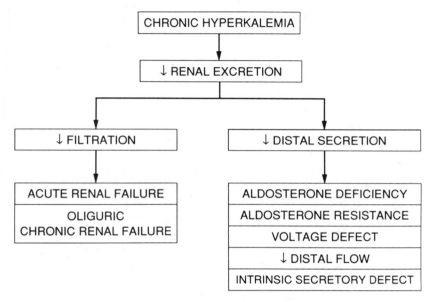

Fig. 4-4. Evaluation of chronic hyperkalemia ($\downarrow$ = decreased).

appear to be excessive. This leaves only two other general mechanisms by which hyperkalemia can develop: a problem with K distribution (internal balance) or a problem with renal K excretion (or both).

Patients with diabetes mellitus have diminished K tolerance,[44] at least in part because of impaired cellular K uptake (e.g., hypoinsulism, hyperglycemia). However, pK rose in the hospital without any overt deterioration in diabetic control (and presumably, therefore, in circulating insulin levels) and in association with a reduction in the blood glucose concentration. The hyperchloremic metabolic acidosis, which may have worsened slightly in the hospital, and the associated alteration in internal K balance,[28] may have contributed to the hyperkalemia but is insufficient to completely account for it. Thus, changes in internal balance do not explain the hyperkalemia in this patient.

Chronic hyperkalemia always implies an inability of the kidneys to remove the excess K[45] (Fig. 4-4). Potassium retention can result from renal failure or from defects in distal tubular K secretion. In *nonoliguric chronic renal failure,* the amount of K secreted per surviving nephron is substantially increased and hyperkalemia usually does not develop until the GFR is less than 10% of normal.[33,46] K retention is much more common in *oliguric chronic renal failure* and *acute renal failure.* The present patient has an estimated GFR of about 45 ml/min; consequently, his hyperkalemia cannot be ascribed to renal insufficiency.

The major factors that modulate distal tubular K secretion are pK (and/or TBK), circulating aldosterone levels, distal tubular flow and distal tubular transepithelial potential difference. It is well known that diabetics, especially those with mild to modest renal insufficiency, have a high incidence of *selective hypoaldosteronism.*[47] This syndrome is characterized by hyperkalemia, hyperchloremic metabolic acidosis, and low circulating renin and aldosterone levels; glucocorticoid function is normal, thus excluding generalized adrenocortical insufficiency (Addison's disease). Diabetes mellitus is by far the most common cause of selective hypoaldosteronism; a variety of chronic tubulointerstitial renal diseases make up most of the remaining cases.[35,47] Although most of these patients have low renin and aldosterone levels, many will also manifest some degree of tubular insensitivity to aldosterone (*pseudohypoaldosteronism*).

2. Which of these causes best explains this patient's current problem?

Selective hypoaldosteronism is certainly an attractive possibility in this patient, but by itself would not explain the abrupt development of hyperkalemia in the hospital. Medications are a common cause of reduced K tolerance,[48] in part by virtue of interfering with the synthesis and/or cellular action of aldosterone. *Nonsteroidal anti-inflammatory agents* impair renin and aldosterone secretion,[49] *angiotensin-converting-enzyme (ACE) inhibitors* block angiotensin II (AII)-mediated aldosterone biosynthesis,[50] *heparin* inhibits adrenal steroidogenesis,[51] and *spironolactone* blocks the renal mineralocorticoid receptor.[52]

In this case, the patient was started on captopril, an ACE inhibitor. Because AII is a potent aldosterone secretogogue, inhibition of AII production would worsen any underlying hypoaldosteronism, thereby precipitating hyperkalemia. Additionally, the low Na diet and fluid restriction that were initiated in the hospital would be expected to reduce distal tubular flow and further limit K secretion. This sequence of events is fairly typical: patients with underlying selective hypoaldosteronism may remain normokalemic until some other factor that further impairs K secretion is introduced. Volume depletion, K-sparing diuretics and ACE inhibitors are common precipitating factors. Given the close association of selective hypoaldosteronism with diabetes mellitus, it is not surprising that defects in internal K balance (e.g., hypoinsulism, hyperglycemia) may also precipitate hyperkalemia in these patients.

3. How would you substantiate the diagnosis?

The diagnosis of selective hypoaldosteronism, and its differentiation from pseudohypoaldosteronism and intrinsic (aldosterone independent) defects in tubular K secretion, can be approached in several ways. The simplest approach is to use renal K excretory capacity as an "assay" of both the presence and the effectiveness of aldosterone. In general, hyperkalemic individuals with normal aldosterone levels and normal mineralocorticoid responsiveness excrete large amounts of K in the urine (urine K concentration >40 mEq/L). Values of less than 20 mEq/L indicate lack of sufficient aldosterone (hypoaldosteronism), lack of aldosterone effect (pseudohypoaldosteronism) or an aldosterone-independent defect in K secretion. Mineralocorticoid replacement will distinguish hypoaldosteronism from the latter two possibilities: Patients with hypoaldosteronism respond with a kaliuresis (and lowering of pK) whereas those with pseudohypoaldosteronism or intrinsic defects in K secretion do not.

Recently, an index that approximates the gradient for distal tubular K secretion (and which may provide more reliable information than the urinary K concentration alone) has been described.[53] The so-called *transtubular K gradient* is calculated as follows: $(U_K/P_K)/(U_{osm}/P_{osm})$, where U_K and P_K are the urine and plasma K concentrations, respectively, and U_{osm} and P_{osm} are the urine and plasma osmolalities, respectively. The index is usually measured before and again 2 hours after an oral dose (0.05 mg) of 9α-fludrocortisone (Florinef), a synthetic mineralocorticoid. A basal value of less than 6 and a stimulated value of greater than 7 are presumptive evidence of hypoaldosteronism and normal tubular responsiveness to mineralocorticoid. Similarly, a value of less than 6 after several days of higher dose Florinef (0.2 mg daily) provides good evidence of mineralocorticoid unresponsiveness.

The definitive diagnosis of selective hypoaldosteronism rests on measuring circulating renin and aldosterone levels (or urinary aldosterone excretion). Under normal circumstances, hyperkalemia increases circulating aldosterone levels.[54] Patients with selective hypoaldosteronism have inappropriately low aldosterone levels despite prevailing hyperkalemia.[35,47,55] Plasma renin activity and plasma aldosterone levels should be measured before and after volume depletion (e.g., low sodium diet) or after the intravenous administration of 40 mg furosemide and 2 hours of upright posture. Under these "stimulated" conditions an increase of less than 3- to 5-fold in plasma renin and aldosterone concentrations is diagnostic of hyporeninemic hypoaldosteronism.

4. How would you treat the hyperkalemia?

A practical approach to immediate therapy in this patient would be to discontinue the captopril and liberalize Na and H_2O intake (watching carefully for any signs of congestive heart failure). The long-term management of patients with selective hypoaldosteronism is challenging.[47] Of utmost importance is the avoidance of situations or therapies that will further exacerbate the already compromised K secretory mechanism, e.g., volume depletion or congestive heart failure (decreased distal tubular flow), ACE inhibitors (drug-induced hypoaldosteronism), spironolactone (drug-induced pseudohypoaldosteronism), and triamterene or amiloride (aldosterone-independent defects in tubular K secretion).

Hormonal replacement may seem to be an ideal therapy, but because mineralocorticoids cause Na retention they are contraindicated in the many patients with selective hypoaldosteronism who have hypertension or congestive heart failure. Oral $NaHCO_3$ (increased distal flow and transepithelial potential difference) is useful in certain situations, but is also limited to patients who can tolerate a high Na intake. Some patients have been successfully treated with a combination of oral $NaHCO_3$ and a loop diuretic, the latter forstalling Na retention and maintaining distal tubular flow. When all else fails, chronic therapy with Kayexalate can be instituted, trying to titrate the amount of the resin to control the hyperkalemia without producing debilitating diarrhea.

CASE STUDY 5

Acute Hyperkalemia Secondary to Rhabdomyolysis

A young man was brought to the emergency room by the police after being found lying in an alley. John Doe was obtunded and hyporeflexic but had no focal neurological signs. Blood pressure was 100/60 mmHg, pulse was 100, and temperature was 96.1°F. He had needle tracks on his arms and legs and multiple ecchymoses and contusions. The remainder of the physical exam was unrevealing. He was given naloxone and dextrose, but showed no improvement in mental status. EKG showed peaked T waves and widening of the QRS.

LABORATORY DATA

Na 150 mEq/L	Glucose 240
K 7.5 mEq/L	BUN 125 mg/dL
Cl 113 mEq/L	Creatinine 17 mg/dL
HCO$_3$ 15 mEq/L	

Arterial blood gas (nasal cannula at 2 L/min): pH 7.30, pCO_2 30, pO_2 180, HCO_3 14
Urinalysis: brown and heme positive
Microscopic exam: 0–3 WBCs and 2–5 RBCs and numerous reddish-brown granular casts

---

Question 1. What do you think happened to Mr. Doe?
Question 2. What are the mechanisms responsible for the hyperkalemia?
Question 3. How would you treat the hyperkalemia in this situation?

1. What do you think happened to Mr. Doe?

The cause of the obtundation is not entirely clear from the information provided. A drug overdose is certainly a possibility (needle tracks), but narcotics have been reasonably excluded (lack of response to the narcotic antagonist, naloxone). Hypoglycemia must always be promptly excluded in any obtunded or comatose patient—hence, the administration of dextrose (again, no response). The lack of focal signs makes a primary neurologic event less likely, but appropriate studies (e.g., CT scan) may be needed for more definitive evaluation of this possibility. Sepsis must always be considered, particularly in drug addicts, and appropriate cultures should be obtained. Finally, it is possible that the obtundation is related to the renal failure (uremia).

The patient has severe renal failure, a decreased BUN/creatinine ratio, an anion gap metabolic acidosis and life-threatening hyperkalemia. The urinalysis is most compatible with acute tubular necrosis (numerous granular casts) and the heme positivity and reddish-brown (heme-stained) casts are typically seen in patients with rhabdomyolysis. The release of myoglobin (a heme-containing muscle protein) and its excretion by the kidney accounts for the heme-positive urine. Myoglobin is thought to act as a direct tubular toxin. A decreased BUN/creatinine ratio is characteristic of the acute renal failure associated with rhabdomyolysis and myoglobinuria. Muscle creatine, when released into the circulation, is oxidized to creatinine; in essence, this represents increased creatinine production and one would therefore expect the serum creatinine concentration to rise out of proportion to the BUN. Elevated serum CPK levels would confirm the suspected diagnosis of rhabdomyolysis.

2. What are the mechanisms responsible for the hyperkalemia?

Let's start with potential changes in external balance. Rhabdomyolysis can be viewed as an endogenous K infusion. If, at the same time, the myoglobinuria causes acute renal failure, you have that most dangerous of situations: K loading (albeit from an endogenous, rather than an exogenous, source) in the face of compromised renal K excretory ability. Hyperkalemia is the predictable result.

Changes in internal balance are probably of lesser importance, but the metabolic acidosis is worthy of mention. Metabolic acidosis is a common concomitant of renal failure; the reduction in renal acid excretion is a result of decreased availability of urinary buffer (decreased ammonia synthesis). As renal acid excretion falls, the inorganic (mineral) acids that are normal end-products of intermediary metabolism (phosphoric, sulfuric acids) accumulate in the body. As this is an inorganic metabolic acidosis, one would expect net redistribution of K out of cells.

3. How would you treat the hyperkalemia in this situation?

Treatment of the hyperkalemia should be directed at: (1) antagonism of the membrane depolarizing effect of hyperkalemia (calcium gluconate), (2) redistribution of K into cells (insulin and glucose, HCO_3), and (3) elimination of K from the body (dialysis). Antagonism and redistribution should be instituted immediately, while preparations for dialysis are made.

CASE STUDY 6

Chronic Hypokalemia and Hypertension

Mr. William Stone, a 25-year-old man with a history of nephrolithiasis, complained of muscle weakness and increased urination over the past few weeks. He was not taking any medications and there was no family history of weakness. Physical exam is completely normal except for mild diffuse muscle weakness.

LABORATORY DATA

Na 138 mEq/L	BUN 18 mg/dL
Cl 110 mEq/L	Creatinine 1.2 mg/dL
K 2.7 mEq/L	WBC 6,500
HCO_3 18 mEq/L	

Urinalysis: pH 6.5, SG 1.005, normal sediment
Arterial blood gas: pH 7.33, pCO_2 34 HCO_3 16
24-hour urine K excretion = 65 mEq.

Question 1. What are the clinical sequelae of hypokalemia?
Question 2. What are the potential causes of hypokalemia in this patient?
Question 3. Which of these potential causes best explain the hypokalemia?

---

1. What are the clinical sequelae of hypokalemia?

Chronic hypokalemia alters cardiac and skeletal muscle function and also has specific renal and endocrinologic effects.[56,57] The best known effect on the heart is a predisposition to digitalis toxicity.[58] However, hypokalemia may also predispose to a wide variety of arrhythmias, especially following myocardial infarction, even in the absence of digitalis therapy.[9,10] The EKG may show flattening of the T wave, ST segment depression and a prominent U wave.[10]

Symptoms related to skeletal muscle dysfunction include malaise, weakness, fatigue, cramps, and the "restless leg" syndrome; tetany, paralysis, and rhabdomyolysis are dramatic manifestations of severe hypokalemia.[59] Hypokalemic periodic paralysis is a rare familial condition in which episodic paralysis is associated with a transient redistribution of K into cells.[60] However, paralysis can be associated with severe hypokalemia of any etiology, especially when pK is less than 2.6 mEq/L.[59] Rhabdomyolysis is usually only seen when pK is less than 3.0 mEq/L, and appears to be due to muscle ischemia (hypokalemia blocks the vasodilation that normally occurs during exercise), as well as to direct effects of hypokalemia on muscle cell metabolism.[59]

Hypokalemia reduces renal blood flow and GFR by altering prostaglandin and AII metabolism.[61] Both renal hypertrophy and chronic interstitial nephritis have been associated with longstanding hypokalemia.[62] Polydipsia and a renal concentrating defect have also been described.[56,62] Primary polydipsia may be related to increased circulating AII levels (AII is a potent dipsogen),[63,64] and the concentrating defect is likely due to a reduction in medullary hypertonicity (possibly because of a defect in chloride transport in the ascending limb of Henle's loop) and alterations in prostaglandin metabolism that reduce the water permeability of the collecting duct.[65] Hypokalemia also increases renal ammoniagenesis[66]; this is particularly important in patients with chronic liver disease in whom hepatic encephalopathy is a common consequence of K depletion.[67] Chronic hypokalemia also promotes metabolic alkalosis. This appears to be due both to increased proximal tubular HCO_3 reabsorption[68] and increased ammonium excretion.[69]

2. What are the potential causes of hypokalemia in this patient?

Although uncommon, *spurious hypokalemia* and *redistribution hypokalemia* should always be considered in the differential diagnosis of the hypokalemic patient. Spurious hypokalemia is due to the ex vivo cellular uptake of K in the setting of severe leukocytosis (WBC > 100,000).[7] Our patient's WBC is only 6,500, so this possibility is excluded. Redistribution hypokalemia is often iatrogenic and therefore obvious. It can also be associated with the rare syndrome of hypokalemic periodic paralysis.[60]

Alkalemia and/or an increase in the plasma HCO_3 concentration can cause mild hypokalemia,[28,29] but a pK as low as 2.7 mEq/L would be unusual and the patient under consideration has a hyperchloremic metabolic acidosis rather than an alkalosis. His plasma HCO_3 concentration is low (rather than high) so he could not have received exogenous HCO_3. Hypokalemia is usually a transient phenomenon in patients who receive excessive amounts of *insulin*.[16] *β-Adrenergic agonists* also enhance cellular K uptake[21] and aerosolized β-agonists (used, for example, by asthmatics) can cause marked hypokalemia and precipitate cardiac arrhythmias.

Poisoning with soluble *barium salts* blocks plasma membrane K channels, impairs the egress of K from cells, and typically presents with vomiting, diarrhea, and severe hypokalemia (pK < 2.0 mEq/L).[70] Inhalation of *toluene* (sniffing paint or glue vapors to induce euphoria) has been associated with severe hypokalemia, muscle weakness, abdominal pain, hematemesis and neuropsychiatric manifestations.[71] Hyperchloremic metabolic acidosis is common and the hypokalemia may be due to renal tubular acidosis, but it has also been suggested that toluene may cause hypokalemia, at least in part, by altering internal K balance.[71] *Hypokalemic periodic paralysis,* a rare autosomal dominant disorder,[60] would be a possibility in this patient if the hypokalemia was epidosic.

If neither spurious nor redistribution hypokalemia is present, the patient must have chronic hypokalemia. As with chronic hyperkalemia, *chronic hypokalemia* implies a problem with external K balance (Fig. 4-5). Because decreased K intake (e.g., anorexia nervosa, "tea and toast" syndrome) is a very unusual sole cause of hypokalemia, the majority of K-depleted patients have

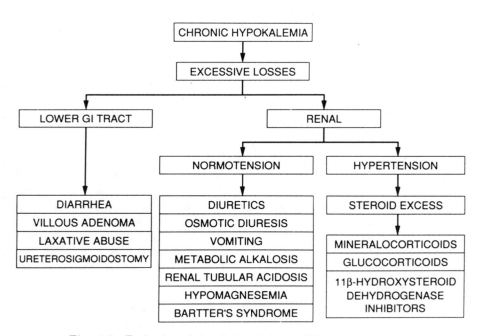

Fig. 4-5. Evaluation of chronic hypokalemia (GI, gastrointestinal).

excessive K losses, either from the lower gastrointestinal tract (e.g., diarrhea, villous adenoma, ureterosigmoidostomy, laxative abuse) or in the urine.

Incorporating information about blood pressure, acid-base status and urinary K excretion is very helpful in developing a differential diagnosis; urinary K excretion should be less than 10 mEq/day in chronically hypokalemic patients with normal renal K handling.[72] The *hypertensive hypokalemic syndromes* (all of which are associated with overproduction of corticosteroids, renal K wasting and oftentimes metabolic alkalosis as well) include primary hyperaldosteronism (e.g., adrenal adenoma, bilateral adrenal hyperplasia), secondary hyperaldosteronism (e.g., renal artery stenosis, malignant hypertension) and Cushing's syndrome (e.g., ACTH-secreting pituitary adenoma, ectopic ACTH syndrome, chronic, high-dose glucocorticoid therapy).

The *normotensive hypokalemic syndromes* are a more heterogeneous group. Excessive fecal K losses are associated with renal K conservation (24-h urinary K excretion <10 mEq), whereas diuretics, osmotic diuresis (e.g., glycosuria), vomiting, certain forms of renal tubular acidosis, hypomagnesemia and Bartter's syndrome are all characterized by renal K wasting (24-h urinary K excretion >20 mEq). Because of the loss of alkali in stool, diarrhea is commonly accompanied by a hyperchloremic metabolic acidosis. So, too, are the renal tubular acidoses. Some causes of renal K wasting are typically associated with metabolic alkalosis (e.g., diuretic use and abuse, vomiting, nasogastric drainage) while others do not present with characteristic alterations in acid-base homeostasis (e.g., hypomagnesemia).

3. Which of these potential causes best explains the hypokalemia?

Our patient's blood pressure is normal, he has a hyperchloremic metabolic acidosis, and is wasting K in the urine. The normal blood pressure excludes states of steroid hormone excess, as does the metabolic acidosis. The prominent renal K wasting excludes lower gastrointestinal K losses, and the absence of metabolic alkalosis excludes surreptitious vomiting.

We are left with the distinct possibility of *renal tubular acidosis* (RTA). The renal tubular acidoses are divided into hypokalemic (proximal RTA and classical distal RTA) and hyperkalemic forms.[73] Proximal RTA is due to impaired proximal bicarbonate reabsorption; the hypokalemia relates to increased delivery of $NaHCO_3$-rich fluid to the distal nephron, Na wasting and secondary hyperaldosteronism. Classical distal RTA is due to an intrinsic defect in distal tubular H^+ secretion. The chronic acidosis inhibits proximal Na reabsorption and promotes urinary Na wasting, which in turn causes secondary hyperaldosteronism. Classical distal RTA is typically associated with hypercalciuria and hypocitraturia (citrate is an important urinary chelator); thus, renal stones are very common.[74] The patient under consideration certainly fits the profile for classical distal RTA.

CASE STUDY 7

Chronic Hypokalemia and Normal Blood Pressure

Miss Cathy Tyler, a 40-year-old woman, was being evaluated for hypertension and fatigue. She has taken hydrochlorothiazide and KCl supplements for the past 2 years. Her blood pressure was 180/105 mmHg without orthostatic changes and her exam was otherwise normal except for mild hyporeflexia.

LABORATORY DATA

Na 140 mEq/L	HCO_3 32 mEq/L
Cl 97 mEq/L	BUN 10 mg/dL
K 2.8 mEq/L	Creatinine 0.8 mg/dL

Review of her laboratory studies before the institution of the diuretic showed K's of 3.0–3.2 mEq/L

EKG: prominent U waves, but otherwise unremarkable

Question 1. What are the potential causes of hypokalemia in this patient and how would you establish the diagnosis?

Question 2. What treatment would you recommend?

---

1. What are the potential causes of hypokalemia in this patient and how would you establish the diagnosis?

Even though the patient takes diuretics, diuretic-induced K depletion is unlikely because she was hypokalemic prior to starting the hydrochlorothiazide. Nonetheless, because essential hypertension and diuretic use (and abuse) are so common, it is always prudent to exclude diuretic-induced K depletion before proceeding to an expensive evaluation for more exotic causes of hypokalemia and hypertension. Measurement of 24-hour urine K excretion would be a sensible next step, but only after the hydrochlorothiazide has been discontinued for several days and Na depletion has been corrected. If necessary, the patient's hypertension can be controlled with agents that do not affect renal K handling (e.g., calcium channel blockers) during this time. This was done, and subsequent tests showed the 24-hour K excretion was 52 mEq at a time when the pK was 2.9 mEq/L. Thus, renal K wasting is documented and the differential diagnosis is narrowed to one of the *hypertensive hypokalemic syndromes* (states of mineralocorticoid or glucocorticoid excess).

In adults, aldosterone is by far the most common mineralocorticoid involved. Aldosterone can either be autonomously produced (*primary hyperaldosteronism*: adrenal adenoma, bilateral adrenal hyperplasia, adrenal carcinoma) or be increased because of high circulating renin levels (*secondary hyperaldosteronism*: renal artery stenosis, malignant hypertension, renin-secreting tumors). Adrenal carcinomas and renin-secreting tumors are exceedingly rare and the patient does not have malignant hypertension. Renal artery stenosis is difficult to exclude on clinical grounds alone—abdominal bruits are not always present and, if there is a serious question of renal artery stenosis (e.g., no other definable cause of the hypokalemia and hypertension), a renal arteriogram should be performed.

Hyperaldosteronism is best documented by measuring plasma aldosterone levels or 24-hour urinary aldosterone excretion after the patient has been on a high Na intake for several days (see reference 81). One potential problem with this approach is that Na loading may exacerbate urinary K wasting and worsen the hypokalemia. Serious hypokalemia can be forstalled by providing K supplements along with the high Na intake. Elevated plasma aldosterone levels or urinary aldosterone excretion (and low plasma renin activity) make the diagnosis of primary hyperaldosteronism.[75] Further evaluation will then be necessary to define the specific cause of the syndrome (*adrenal adenoma, adrenal hyperplasia* or *adrenal carcinoma*).[75,76]

If both renin and aldosterone are suppressed, an unidentified mineralocorticoid must be present. For example, glycyrrhizic acid, a component of unprocessed licorice, inhibits 11β-hydroxysteroid dehydrogenase, a renal enzyme that rapidly inactivates cortisol.[77] In the absence of 11β-hydroxysteroid dehydrogenase activity, prevailing renal cortisol levels are easily able to activate the mineralocorticoid receptor (see reference 83). Carbenoxalone, a derivative of glycyrrhetinic acid, is used in Europe for therapy of peptic ulcer disease. It, too, inhibits 11β-hydroxysteroid dehydrogenase activity, resulting in hypokalemia.

If both renin and aldosterone levels are elevated, a primary increase in renin production (e.g., *renal artery stenosis, malignant hypertension, renin-secreting tumor*) have to be considered. With renovascular disease, reduced renal blood flow increases renin production in the relatively ischemic kidney. Increased circulating AII levels mediate the hypertension, and the resulting secondary hyperaldosteronism mediates the renal K wasting.

Interestingly, patients with congestive heart failure and secondary hyperaldosteronism do not commonly manifest hypokalemia unless treated with diuretics. This is because the decreased renal blood flow reduces distal tubular flow, thus limiting K secretion despite high circulating aldosterone levels. Diuretic therapy enhances distal delivery and in the face of prevailing hyperaldosteronism leads to marked kaliuresis. This can be put to use diagnostically in patients with suspected hyperaldosteronism. Patients with primary hyperaldosteronism will manifest increased K wasting and hypokalemia when placed on a high Na intake, but patients with secondary hyperaldosteronism will tend to suppress renin and aldosterone production and not waste K.

2. What treatment would you recommend?

The patient under consideration was found to have inappropriately elevated urinary K excretion despite marked hypokalemia, suppressed plasma renin activity and an increased plasma aldosterone level. A CT scan showed no evidence of an adrenal tumor. The best way to differentiate between a small (<1 cm^2) adrenal tumor that could be missed on CT scan (which occurs in 15%–25% of adrenal adenomas) and bilateral adrenal hyperplasia is by selective adrenal vein sampling. Adrenal vein plasma aldosterone levels did not lateralize in our patient, indicating the presence of bilateral adrenal hyperplasia. This is best treated with the aldosterone receptor blocker, spironolactone.[78,79] Other K-sparing diuretics that have been successfully used are amiloride and triamterene. The patient was treated with amiloride. Her blood pressure was kept in good control, and the hypokalemia was resolved. If the patient had an adrenal adenoma rather than adrenal hyperplasia, surgical removal of the tumor would be the appropriate therapy.

CASE STUDY 8

Chronic Hypokalemia and Normal Blood Pressure

Ms. Ann Moreau, a 25-year-old female with a history of irritable bowel syndrome, was evaluated for frequent bowel movements. Her physical exam was completely normal, and the stool was heme negative and contained no WBCs.

LABORATORY DATA

Na 135 mEq/L	HCO_3 32 mEq/L
Cl 95 mEq/L	BUN 10 mg/dL
K 3.0 mEq/L	Creatinine 0.6 mg/dL

Question 1. What is the cause of hypokalemia in this patient and how would you establish the diagnosis?

Question 2. How would you treat the patient?

---

1. What is the cause of hypokalemia in this patient and how would you establish the diagnosis?

In patients with chronic hypokalemia and normal blood pressure, steroid excess is unlikely. As usual, the initial step in the evaluation will be a good history, with particular attention in this case to surreptitious vomiting and to diuretic and/or laxative abuse. If this is unrevealing, the 24-hour urine K excretion will define whether renal or lower gastrointestinal K wasting is present. Consideration of the acid-base status will also be very helpful.

Colonic losses of alkaline salts are common in patients with *diarrhea,* who typically present with hypokalemia and hyperchloremic metabolic acidosis.[80] *Chronic laxative abuse* (often surreptitious) can be associated with marked hypokalemia, even in the absence of overt diarrhea.[81] Although hyperchloremic metabolic acidosis may occur with chronic laxative abuse, it is not unusual to see metabolic alkalosis in those patients with concomitant Na (volume) depletion and secondary hyperaldosteronism.[82] *Villous adenoma* of the rectum also presents with a variable acid-base pattern, which depends on the relative rates of HCO_3 and Cl secretion by the tumor.[83] *Chronic diuretic abuse* (also often surreptitious) is typically associated with metabolic alkalosis.[84] *Surreptitious vomiting* is another common cause of hypokalemia and metabolic alkalosis. The loss of HCl generates the alkalosis and secondary hyperaldosteronism, bicarbonaturia, and increased distal tubular flow account for the K wasting.[85]

On an ad lib Na and K intake, the patient was found to have a 24-hour urinary K excretion of 62 mEq at a time when pK was 3.3 mEq/L; repeat arterial blood gases showed a persistent metabolic alkalosis. Pursuing the cause of the metabolic alkalosis is often revealing in such patients. The first step is a urinary Cl determination since a urinary Cl excretion of less than 10 mEq/day suggests gastric fluid loss (e.g., surreptitious vomiting) and a urinary Cl excretion of greater than 10 mEq/day suggests diuretic abuse, Mg depletion, or Bartter's syndrome.

Magnesium depletion is associated with renal K wasting, hypokalemia, and hypocalcemia. The mechanisms underlying the K wasting are unknown but the urinary K losses resolve promptly following Mg repletion.[86] Magnesium depletion is more common than previously recognized, especially in chronic alcoholics and in patients taking diuretics (which induce both K and Mg wasting; the resulting Mg depletion exacerbates the kaliuresis). The plasma Mg concentration should always be checked in patients with otherwise unexplained hypokalemia.

Bartter's syndrome is characterized by hypokalemia, metabolic alkalosis and normal blood pressure (despite hyperplasia of the juxtaglomerular apparatus and activation of the renin-angiotensin-aldosterone system).[87] The exact cause of this disorder remains to be delineated, but abnormalities in renal prostaglandin metabolism and a defect in loop of Henle Cl transport have been implicated.[88,89]

The urinary Cl concentration in the patient under consideration was 35 mEq/day, implicating diuretics as a likely cause of the hypokalemia and metabolic alkalosis. The plasma Mg concentration was borderline low. Surreptitious diuretic use is a common cause of hypokalemia and metabolic alkalosis in young women concerned about their weight and can be confirmed by sending a urine sample for diuretic drug analysis. If diuretic abuse is definitively excluded, serious consideration would have to be given to Bartter's syndrome.

2. How would you treat the patient?

Repletion of K stores requires estimation of the magnitude of the deficit and determination of whether continuing losses are expected. Unfortunately, pK does not always reflect the extent of the associated total body K deficit because many factors modulate pK, thereby altering internal K balance independently of changes in total body K.[29] When hypokalemia is uncomplicated by any factors that acutely affect internal K balance, pK decreases by approximately 0.3 mEq/L for each decrement of 100 mEq total body K.[29] Thus, it is likely that the present patient has a total body K deficit of at least 500 mEq.

Asymptomatic hypokalemia is best treated with oral K replacement. KCl should be employed in the presence of Cl depletion and metabolic alkalosis. There are few well-defined guidelines for the proper oral dosing of K, but a single oral dose should probably not exceed the hourly intravenous dose (used in more life-threatening situations): 0.6 mEq/kg in patients with normal renal function, 0.3 mEq/kg in patients with renal insufficiency and 0.1 to 0.2 mEq/kg in patients with diabetes mellitus, depending on their renal function.[8,90]

The patient under consideration weighed 55 kg. Thus, 30 mEq 3 times a day for several days should suffice to bring pK back into a safe range. The provision of a normal diet, stopping the diuretic use, and appropriate counselling or psychotherapy would also be indicated.

REFERENCES

1. Romano AT, Young GR Jr: Mild forearm exercise during venipuncture and its effect on potassium determinations. Clin Chem 2:303, 1977
2. Mather A, Mackie NR: Effects of hemolysis on serum electrolyte values. Clin Chem 6:223, 1960
3. Ingram RH Jr, Seki M: Pseudohyperkalemia with thrombocytosis. N Engl J Med 267:895, 1962
4. Bronson WR, DeVita VT, Carbone PP et al: Pseudohyperkalemia due to release of potassium from white blood cells during clotting. N Engl J Med 274:369, 1966
5. Ho-Yen DO, Pennington CR: Pseudohyperkalemia and infectious mononucleosis. Postgrad Med 556: 435, 1980
6. James DR, Stansbie D: Familial pseudohyperkalemia: Inhibition of erythrocyte K^+ efflux at 4°C by quinine. Clin Sci 73:557, 1987
7. Adams PC, Woodhouse KSW, Adela M et al: Exaggerated hypokalemia in acute myeloid leukemia. Br Med J 282:1034, 1981
8. Sterns RH, Guzzo J, Feig PU: The disposition of intravenous potassium in normal man: the role of insulin. Clin Sci 61:23, 1981
9. Epstein FH: Signs and symptoms of electrolyte disorders. p. 499. In Maxwell MH, Kleeman CR (eds): Clinical Disorders of Fluid and Electrolyte Metabolism. 3rd Ed. McGraw Hill, New York, 1980
10. Surawicz B: Relationship between electrocardiogram and electrolytes. Am Heart J 73:814, 1967
11. Szerlip H, Weiss J, Singer I: Profound hyperkalemia without electrocardiographic changes. Am J Kid Dis 7:461, 1986

12. Chamberlain MJ: Emergency treatment of hyperkalemia. Lancet 1:464, 1964
13. Braun HA, Van Horne R, Bettinger C, Bellet S: The influence of hypocalcemia induced by sodium ethylendiamine acetate on the toxicity of potassium: an experimental study. J Lab Clin Med 46:544, 1955
14. Shrager MW: Digitalis intoxication. Arch Intern Med 100:881, 1957
15. Zierler KL, Rabinowitz D: Effect of very small concentrations of insulin on forearm metabolism: persistence of its action on potassium and free fatty acids without its effects on glucose. J Clin Invest 43:950, 1964
16. DeFronzo RA, Felig P, Ferrannini E, Wahren J: Effect of graded doses of insulin on splanchnic and peripheral potassium metabolism in man. Am J Physiol 238:E421, 1980
17. Goldfarb S, Cox M, Singer I, Goldberg M: Acute hyperkalemia induced by hyperglycemia: hormonal mechanisms. Ann Intern Med 84:426, 1976
18. Fraley DS, Adler S: Isohydric regulation of plasma potassium by bicarbonate in the rat. Kidney Int 9:333, 1976
19. Fraley DS, Adler S: Correction of hyperkalemia by bicarbonate despite constant blood pH. Kidney Int 12:354, 1977
20. Blumberg A, Weidmann P, Shaw S, Gnadinger M: Effect of various therapeutic approaches on plasma potassium and major regulating factors in terminal renal failure. Am J Med 85:507, 1988
21. Clausen T, Flatman JA: Beta$_2$-adrenoceptors mediate the stimulating effect of adrenaline on active electrogenic Na-K-transport in rat soleus muscle. Br J Pharmacol 68:749, 1980
22. Montouliu J, Lens KL, Revert L: Potassium lowering effect of albuterol for hyperkalemia in renal failure. Arch Intern Med 147:713, 1987
23. Wang P, Clausen T: Treatment of attacks of hyperkalemic familial periodic paralysis by inhalation of salbutamol. Lancet 1:221, 1976
24. Flinn RB, Merrill JP, Welzant WR: Treatment of the oliguric patient with a new sodium polysterene resin and sorbitol. N Engl J Med 264:111, 1961
25. Sebastian A, Schambelan M: Amelioration of hyperchloremic acidosis with furosemide therapy in patients with chronic renal insufficiency and type IV renal tubular acidosis. Am J Nephrol 4:287, 1984
26. Brown ST, Ahearn DJ, Nolph KD: Potassium removal with peritoneal dialysis. Kidney Int 4:67, 1973
27. Santusanio F, Faloona GF, Knochel JP et al: Evidence for a role of endogenous insulin and glucagon in the regulation of potassium homeostasis. J Lab Clin Med 81:809, 1973
28. Adrogue HJ, Madias NE: Changes in plasma potassium concentration during acute acid-base disturbances. Am J Med 71:456, 1981
29. Sterns RH, Cox M, Feig PU et al: Internal potassium balance and the control of the plasma potassium concentration. Medicine 60:339, 1981
30. Oster JR, Perez GO, Castra A et al: Plasma potassium response to acute metabolic acidosis induced by mineral and nonmineral acids. Mineral Electrolyte Metab 4:28, 1980
31. Orringer CE, Eustace JC, Wunsch CD et al: Natural history of lactic acidosis after grand-mal seizures. N Engl J Med 297:796, 1977
32. Fulop M: Serum potassium in lactic acidosis and ketoacidosis. N Engl J Med 300:1087, 1979
33. Von Ypersele de Strihou C: Potassium homeostasis in renal failure. Kidney Int 11:491, 1977
34. Molitch ME, Rodman E, Hirsch CA, Dubinsky E: Spurious serum creatinine elevations in ketoacidosis. Ann Intern Med 93:280, 1980
35. Schambelan M, Sebastian A, Biglieri EG: Prevalence pathogenesis and functional significance of aldosterone deficiency in hyperkalemic patients with chronic renal insufficiency. Kidney Int 17:89, 1980
36. Gennari FJ, Kassirer JP: Osmotic diuresis. N Engl J Med 291:714, 1974
37. Adrogue HJ, Lederer Ed, Suki WN, Eknoyan G: Determinants of plasma potassium levels in diabetic ketoacidosis. Medicine 65:163, 1986
38. Biegelman PM: Potassium in severe diabetic ketoacidosis. Am J Med 54:419, 1973
39. Fulop M: The treatment of severely uncontrolled diabetes mellitus. Adv Intern Med 25:327, 1984
40. Illingworth RN, Proudfoot AT: Rapid poisoning with slow release potassium. Br Med J 2:485, 1980
41. Moss MH, Rasen AR: Potassium toxicity due to intravenous penicillin therapy. Pediatrics 29:1032, 1962

42. Bay WH, Hartman JA: High potassium in low sodium soups (letter). N Engl J Med 308:1166, 1983
43. Schwartz WB: Potassium and the kidney. N Engl J Med 253:601, 1955
44. DeFronzo RA, Sherwin RS, Dillingham M et al: Influence of basal insulin and glucagon secretion on potassium and sodium metabolism: studies with somatostatin in normal dogs and in normal and diabetic human beings. J Clin Invest 61:472, 1978
45. Rose BD: Clinical Physiology of Acid-Base and Electrolyte Disorders. 3rd Ed. McGraw-Hill, New York, 1989
46. Schultze RG, Taggart DD, Shapiro H et al: On the adaptation in potassium excretion associated with nephron reduction in the dog. J Clin Invest 50:1061, 1971
47. DeFronzo RA: Hyperkalemia and hyporeninemic hypoaldosteronism. Kidney Int 17:118, 1980
48. Ponce SP, Jennings AE, Madias NE, Harrington JT: Drug-Induced hyperkalemia. Medicine 64:357, 1985
49. Kutyrina IM, Androsova SO, Warshavski VA et al: Effects of indomethacin on the renal function and renin-aldosterone system in chronic glomerulonephritis. Nephron 32:244, 1982
50. Atlas SA, Case DB, Sealey JE et al: Interruption of the renin-angiotensin system in hypertensive patients by captopril induces sustained reduction in aldosterone secretion, potassium retention and natriuresis. Hypertension 1:274, 1979
51. Sherman RA, Ruddy MC: Suppression of aldosterone production by low dose heparin. Am J Nephrol 6:165, 1986
52. Corvol P, Claire M, Oblin ME et al: Mechanism of the anti-mineralcorticoid effects of spironolactone. Kidney Int 20:1, 1981
53. West ML, Marsden PA, Richardson RM et al: New clinical approach to evaluate disorders of potassium excretion. Mineral Electrolyte Metab 12:234, 1986
54. Douglas JG: Effects of high potassium diet on angiotensin II receptors and angiotensin induced aldosterone production in rat adrenal glomerular cells. Endocrinology 106:983, 1980
55. Schambelan M, Stockigt JR, Biglieri EG: Isolated hypoaldosteronism in adults: a renin-deficiency syndrome. New Engl J Med 287:573, 1972
56. Manitius A, Levitan H, Beck D, Epstein F: On the mechanism of impairment of renal concentrating ability in potassium deficiency. J Clin Invest 39:684, 1960
57. Helderman JH, Elahi D, Anderson DK et al: Prevention of the glucose intolerance of thiazide diuretics by maintenance of the body potassium. Diabetes 32:106, 1983
58. Shapiro W, Taubert K: Hypokalemia and digoxin-induced arrhythmias. Lancet 2:604, 1975
59. Knochel JP: Neuromuscular manifestations of electrolyte disorders. Am J Med 75:521, 1982
60. Layzer RB: Periodic paralysis and the sodium-potassium pump. Ann Neurol 11:547, 1982
61. Linas SL, Dickmann D: Mechanism of the decreased renal blood flow in the potassium-depleted conscious rat. Kidney Int 21:757, 1982
62. Schwartz WB, Relman AS: Effects of electrolyte disorders on renal structure and function. N Engl J Med 276:383, 1967
63. Yamamoto T, Shimizu M, Morioka M et al: Role of angiotensin II in the pathogenesis of hyperdipsia in chronic renal failure. JAMA 256:604, 1986
64. Saikaley A, Bichet D, Kucharcyzk J et al: Neuroendocrine factors mediating polydipsia induced by dietary Na, Cl, and K depletion. Am J Physiol 251:R1071, 1986
65. Eknoyan G, Martinez-Maldonado M, Suki WN et al: Renal diluting capacity in the hypokalemic rat. Am J Physiol 219:933, 1970
66. Tannen RL: Relationship of renal ammonia production and potassium homeostasis. Kidney Int 11:453, 1977
67. Baertl JM, Sancetta SM, Gabuzda GH: Relation of acute potassium depletion to renal ammonium metabolism in patients with cirrhosis. J Clin Invest 42:696, 1963
68. Capasso G, Kinne R, Malnic G et al: Renal bicarbonate reabsorption in the rat: Effects of hypokalemia and carbonic anhydrase. J Clin Invest 78:1558, 1986
69. Tannen RL: Effect of potassium on renal acidification and acid-base homeostasis. Sem Nephrol 7:263, 1987

70. Roza O, Berman LB: The pathophysiology of barium: Hypokalemic and cardiovascular effects. J Pharmacol Exp Ther 177:433, 1971
71. Streicher HZ, Gabow PA, Moss AH et al: Syndromes of toluene sniffing in adults. Ann Intern Med 94:758, 1981
72. Squires RD, Huth EJ: Experimental potassium depletion in normal human subjects. I. Relation of ionic intakes to the renal conservation of potassium. J Clin Invest 38:1134, 1959
73. Davidman M, Schmitz P: Renal tubular acidosis. a pathophysiologic approach. Hospital Practice p. 77. January 30, 1988
74. Coe FL, Parks JH: Stone disease in hereditary distal renal tubular acidosis. Ann Intern Med 93:60, 1980
75. Bravo EL, Tarazi RC, Dustan HP et al: The changing clinical spectrum of primary aldosteronism. Am J Med 74:641, 1983
76. Nath RH, Biglieri EG: Primary hyperaldosteronism. Med Clin NA 72:1117, 1988
77. Funder JW, Pearce PT, Smith R, Smith AI. Mineralocorticoid action. Target tissue specificity is enzyme, not receptor mediated. Science 242:583, 1988
78. Weinberger MH, Grim CE, Hollifield JW et al: Primary aldosteronism. Diagnosis, localization and treatment. Ann Intern Med 90:386, 1979
79. Ganguly A, Donohue JP: Primary aldosteronism: pathophysiology, diagnosis, and treatment. J Urol 129:241, 1979
80. Editorial. Diarrhea and acid-base disturbances. Lancet 1:1305, 1966
81. Schwartz WB, Relman AS: Metabolic and renal studies in chronic potassium depletion resulting from overuse of laxatives. J Clin Invest 32:258, 1953
82. Fleming BJ, Genuth SM, Gouls AB et al: Laxative induced hypokalemia, sodium depletion and hyperreninemia. Ann Intern Med 83:60, 1975
83. Shnitka TK, Freidman MHW, Kidd EG et al: Villous tumors of the rectum and colon characterized by severe fluid and electrolyte loss. Surg Gynecol Obstet 112:609, 1961
84. Schwartz WB, von Ypersele de Strihou C, Kassirer JP: Role of anions in metabolic alkalosis and potassium deficiency. N Engl J Med 279:630, 1968
85. Needle MA, Kaloyanides GJ, Schwartz WB: The effects of selective depletion of hydrochloric acid on acid-base and electrolyte equilibrium. J Clin Invest 43:1836, 1964
86. Whang R, Flink EB, Dyckner T et al: Magnesium depletion as a cause of refractory potassium repletion. Arch Intern Med 145:1686, 1985
87. Bartter FC, Pronove P, Gill JR Jr et al: Hyperplasia of the juxtaglomerular complex with hyperaldosteronism and hypokalemic alkalosis. A new syndrome. Am J Med 33:811, 1962
88. Fichman MP, Telfer N, Zia P et al: Role of prostaglandins in the pathogenesis of Bartter's syndrome. Am J Med 60:785, 1976
89. Gill JR Jr: The role of chloride transport in the thick ascending limb in the pathogenesis of Bartter's syndrome. Klin Wochensch 60:1212, 1982
90. Kruse JA, Carlson RW: Rapid correction of hypokalemia using concentrated intravenous potassium chloride infusions. Arch Intern Med 150:613, 1990

5

Metabolic Acidosis

Fuad Shihab
Fuad N. Ziyadeh

PATHOPHYSIOLOGY

Normal Range of Blood pH

The normal range of blood pH is 7.38 to 7.42 and represents the negative decimal logarithm of the hydrogen ion concentration. Acidemia signifies an increase in blood hydrogen ion concentration above 40 nEq/L (10^{-9} Eq/L) or a decrease in blood pH below 7.38. This can be initiated by either an increase in $PaCO_2$ or a decrease in bicarbonate concentration. When a decrease in bicarbonate concentration initiates the disturbance, it is called metabolic acidosis. Metabolic acidosis is produced either by the addition of a nonvolatile acid from endogenous or exogenous sources, or by the loss of alkali from the kidney or gastrointestinal tract.

Body Response to Acidosis

The response of the body to an increase in hydrogen ion concentration involves three processes: (1) buffering (extracellular and intracellular), (2) respiratory compensation, and (3) renal excretion of the H^+ load, which represents the definitive correction. Figure 5-1 illustrates the time course of the three phases of defense against an acid load.

Buffering

This is the first line of defense that minimizes the changes in H^+ concentration. It occurs almost immediately (minutes to hours) after the addition of the H^+ ions.

Extracellular Buffering

The carbonic acid-bicarbonate buffer system is quantitatively the most important buffer in the extracellular fluid. This system is amenable to homeostatic regulation by the dual control of pulmonary function (regulation of $PaCO_2$) and renal function (regulation of serum HCO_3^-). The following equations are used to describe the equilibrium state of this buffer system in the blood.

Henderson equation

$$[H^+](nEq/L) = 24 \times (PaCO_2/[HCO_3^-]) \qquad \text{(Eq. 5-1)}$$

97

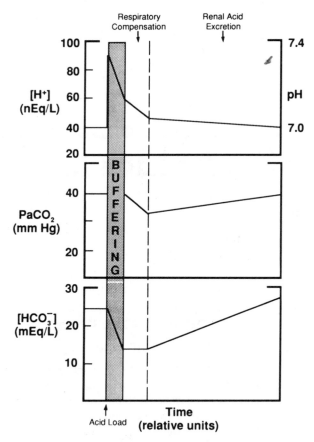

Fig. 5-1. Schematic representation of the three phases of defense against an acid load: buffering, respiratory compensation, and definitive correction (renal acid excretion).

Henderson-Hasselbalch equation

$$pH = 6.1 + \log[HCO_3^-]/0.3\ PaCO_2 \qquad \text{(Eq. 5-2)}$$

The ability of this buffer system to prevent large changes in the blood pH is illustrated in the following example. If the normal $PaCO_2$ is 40 mmHg and the normal plasma HCO_3^- concentration is 24 mEq/L, then the normal H^+ ion concentration is $[H^+] = 24 \times 40/24 = 40$ nEq/L, which corresponds to a pH of 7.40. Let us assume that 12 mEq of H^+ are added to each liter of extracellular fluid. If the bicarbonate buffer system was not present, the H^+ concentration would have increased from 40 to 160 nEq/L, which corresponds to a pH of 6.8. However, as H^+ is added to the plasma it is buffered by HCO_3^-. The plasma HCO_3^- concentration will fall from 24 to 12 mEq/L. The corresponding H^+ ion concentration will then be $[H^+] = 24 \times 40/12 = 80$ nEq/L which corresponds to a pH of only 7.10.

Intracellular Buffering

Hydrogen ions are also able to enter the cells and be taken up by the intracellular buffers (hemoglobin, proteins, and phosphates) and bone buffers. Approximately 55% to 60% of an acid load is buffered by the cells and bone within a few hours. As a result, the addition of 12 mEq of H^+ per liter of extracellular fluid will actually lower the plasma HCO_3^- concentration by only 5 mEq/L instead of 12 mEq/L.

Respiratory Compensation

In addition to buffering, the change in blood pH is also limited acutely by respiratory compensation. Acidemia, through its action on central and peripheral chemoreceptors, stimulates alveolar hyperventilation. This increase in ventilation begins within 1 to 2 hours and reaches its maximum level at 12 to 24 hours. This will tend to lower the $PaCO_2$ and, accordingly, will bring the blood pH toward normal. Respiratory compensation does not, however, completely correct the pH. Therefore, H^+ concentration will approach but not quite reach the normal range.

The application of Winters' formula, derived empirically from clinical conditions characterized by uncomplicated, simple metabolic acidosis, is helpful in estimating the appropriateness of the respiratory compensation to metabolic acidosis [expected $PaCO_2 = (1.5 \times HCO_3^-) + 8 \pm 2$]. If the calculated $PaCO_2$ is close to that of the recommended $PaCO_2$, it implies that the prevailing acid-base disturbance represents a single event comprised of metabolic acidosis with the associated appropriate respiratory compensation.

Renal H^+ Handling

The kidneys provide the mechanism for the correction of metabolic acidosis, the third and final line of defense against acidification of body fluids. As shown in Figure 5-1, the kidneys are responsible for increasing the serum HCO_3^- back to normal values. To better understand this, we will review briefly the renal handling of HCO_3^- and H^+ ions.

The kidneys are actively involved in maintaining acid-base balance and keeping the blood pH at about 7.40. To do this, there are two functions that must be performed by the kidney: (1) the filtered bicarbonate must be reabsorbed, and (2) the daily production of metabolically generated H^+ must be removed from the body (normally 1 mEq/kg derived from oxidation of dietary protein and nucleotides). The kidney generates new bicarbonate, which is added to the blood in order to replenish the bicarbonate that is buffered by the H^+ ions produced by metabolic processes.

Bicarbonate Reclamation

Bicarbonate is freely filterable at the glomerulus. At normal plasma levels (24 mEq/L), 4800 mEq/day are filtered and would be lost in the urine unless reabsorption occurred. The proximal tubule accounts for reclamation of more than 90 percent of filtered bicarbonate. The mechanism for this process is shown in Figure 5-2; H^+ is secreted largely by a Na^+/H^+ exchanger on the luminal brush-border membrane. In the tubular lumen, the H^+ reacts with the filtered HCO_3^- to form H_2CO_3, which is dehydrated to CO_2 and H_2O. This latter reaction is catalyzed by carbonic anhydrase present on the luminal brush border membrane. Carbon dioxide diffuses passively into the cell. Within the cell, H_2O is split to yield the H^+ which is secreted in the tubular lumen and OH^-, which reacts with CO_2 in a carbonic anhydrase catalyzed reaction to yield HCO_3^-. The HCO_3^- is then transported to the blood along with Na^+ ions at the basolateral border of proximal tubular cells in a Na^+/HCO_3^- cotransport mechanism. The cortical and medullary collecting ducts are responsible for reclaiming the remaining 10% of filtered HCO_3^-.

Bicarbonate Generation

The distal nephron is responsible not only for reclaiming the remaining filtered HCO_3^- but is also the site of excretion of the dietary acid load generated daily. Hydrogen is secreted by an active H^+-ATPase pump located at the luminal border of the intercalated cells (Fig. 5-2). The rate at which H^+ is secreted is influenced by several factors, including the potential difference

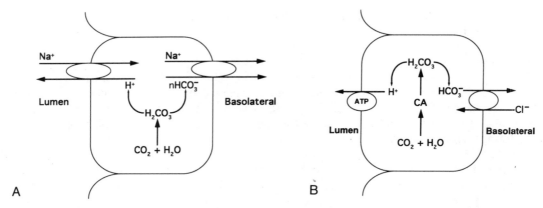

Fig. 5-2. General mechanisms for H^+ and HCO_3^- transport across the apical and basolateral membranes of (**A**) a proximal renal tubule cell and (**B**) a distal renal tubule cell.

across the tubular cell and aldosterone. Sodium reabsorption by the neighboring principal cells generates, a negative lumen potential, which enhances the rate of the H^+ secretory pump. Aldosterone also increases the rate of H^+ secretion. Aldosterone action to stimulate H^+ secretion occurs at multiple sites: stimulation of Na^+ reabsorption in the collecting duct, thus increasing lumen negativity; stimulation of NH_3 production by aldosterone-induced hypokalemia; and, perhaps, through a direct effect of the hormone to increase H^+ pump activity. The secreted H^+ reacts with urinary buffers (most notably, NH_3 and phosphates). A portion of the secreted H^+ also reacts with the filtered HCO_3^- to form H_2CO_3, which is dehydrated to CO_2 and H_2O.

Net Acid Excretion
Net acid excretion (NAE) refers to the net amount of H^+ removed from the body by renal excretion in a given period of time. In a healthy person, the NAE equals the daily metabolic production of acid. If some HCO_3^- is also lost from the body through the urine, this will lead to the net addition of H^+ to body fluids. Therefore, NAE is calculated as follows:

$$NAE = (U\ NH_4^+ \times V) + (U\ TA \times V) - (U\ HCO_3^- \times V) \qquad \text{(Eq. 5-3)}$$

$$\text{where } U \times V = \text{urinary excretion; } TA = \text{titrable acids}$$

The most important urinary buffer is NH_3, because it allows for the excretion of more than 60% of the daily nonvolatile acid load. Additionally, renal production of NH_3 is under fine homeostatic control; it can be increased by up to 10-fold if net acid excretion is also increased. This allows for excretion of large amounts of acid in situations of increased acid production. In contrast, excretion of H^+ as titrable acids (TA) is constant at around 30 mEq/day and is limited by filtration and reabsorption of phosphates. Ammonia is produced largely by deamidation and deamination of glutamine in the proximal tubule. It enters the tubular fluid by passive diffusion and reacts with H^+ in the lumen to form NH_4^+, which diffuses minimally and thus is trapped in the lumen. The buffering of the secreted H^+ by NH_3 prevents a fall in pH in the lumen below 4.5 to 5.0, which allows the rate of H^+ secretion to continue without development of a more unfavorable cell-to-lumen H^+ gradient. Following an acid load, the kidney requires a lag period of 3 to 4 days before it reaches its maximum level of H^+ excretion.

CLINICAL FEATURES

Hyperventilation (Kussmaul Respiration)

The presence of deep, rhythmic respirations is induced by stimulation of the respiratory center in the brain stem by the low blood pH.

Hypotension

Hypotension may also be observed in severely acidemic patients. This hemodynamic compromise is the result of depressed myocardial contractility and arterial vasodilatation, both induced by a severely low blood pH (below 7.20). Ventricular arrhythmias may also develop.

Gastrointestinal Disturbance

The patient may also manifest nonspecific gastrointestinal symptoms, including anorexia, nausea and vomiting. By causing the loss of H^+ ions from the body, vomiting may actually be protective.

Hyperkalemia

Hyperkalemia occurs mostly in the setting of inorganic acidoses like renal failure (retention of sulfuric and phosphoric acids) or exogenous HCl administration. The genesis of this hyperkalemia remains unclear but it is assumed to result from transcellular shifts of potassium in exchange for H^+ which enters the cells to be buffered by intracellular buffers. This shift does not appear to occur with organic acidoses, such as lactic acidosis and ketoacidosis.

Osteopenia

When metabolic acidosis becomes longstanding, skeletal manifestations such as osteopenia begin to manifest. Growth retardation is observed in children with renal failure or renal tubular acidosis.

DIFFERENTIAL DIAGNOSIS

Many disorders can cause metabolic acidosis. From a diagnostic viewpoint, calculation of the anion gap (AG) is helpful in dividing metabolic acidosis into two major types: (1) acidosis with a normal AG (also called hyperchloremic), and (2) acidosis with an increased AG (also called normochloremic).

Anion Gap

Electroneutrality demands that the number of positive charges equals the number of negative charges contained on ions and macromolecules in the serum (that is, mEq of cations equal mEq of anions).

$$Na^+ + K^+ + Ca^{2+} + Mg^{2+} = Cl^- + HCO_3^- + HPO_4^{2-} + OA^- + PR^- + SO_4^{2-} \quad \text{(Eq. 5-4)}$$

$$\text{where OA} = \text{organic anions and PR} = \text{proteins}$$

Not all of these moieties are routinely measured in the clinical laboratory. By convention, we call Na^+, Cl^-, and HCO_3^- the measured ions. The above equation may be simplified by calling

K^+, Ca^{++}, and Mg^{++} unmeasured cations (UC^+) and HPO_4^{2-}, OA^-, SO_4^{2-}, and PR^- unmeasured anions (UA^-):

$$Na^+ + UC^+ = Cl^- + HCO_3^- + UA^- \qquad \text{(Eq. 5-5)}$$

The anion gap represents the difference between the concentration of unmeasured anions and cations.

$$\text{Anion gap (mEq/L)} = [UA^-] - [UC^+] \qquad \text{(Eq. 5-6)}$$

By rearrangement of the above equations the anion gap can be calculated as follows:

$$\text{Anion gap (mEq/L)} = [Na^+] - ([Cl^-] + [HCO_3^-]) \qquad \text{(Eq. 5-7)}$$

The normal AG is 12 ± 4 mEq/L. The negative charges on the plasma proteins (mostly albumin) account for most of the anion gap. For the most part, increases in AG almost always signify a subtype of metabolic acidosis that is referred to as high AG metabolic acidosis.

Increased Anion Gap (Normochloremic)

High AG metabolic acidosis is associated with reduced serum bicarbonate because of buffering by an added H^+ ion. In addition, an unmeasured anion (such as lactate or beta hydroxybutyrate) is retained with the added H^+. This leads to an elevation of the AG. In this case, the concentration of Cl^- remains virtually unchanged.

The major causes of metabolic acidosis with an elevated anion gap (Table 5-1) are ketoacidosis, lactic acidosis, renal failure, and ingestion of toxins. Mild elevation of the anion gap (AG < 20

Table 5-1.   Differential Diagnosis of Metabolic Acidosis

High Anion Gap (Normochloremic)	Normal Anion Gap (Hyperchloremic)

Increased acid production
  Lactic acidosis
  Ketoacidosis
    Diabetic
    Alcoholic
    Starvation
	Gastrointestinal losses of bicarbonate
	  Diarrhea
	  Small bowel or pancreatic drainage and fistula
	  Ureterosigmoidostomy, long or obstructed
	    ileal loop or conduit
	  Anion exchange resins
	  Ingestion of $CaCl_2$, $MgCl_2$

Ingestion of toxic substances
  Salicylate
  Methanol
  Ethylene glycol
  Others (paraldehyde, toluene)
	Renal losses of bicarbonate
	  Proximal (type 2) RTA
	  Carbonic anhydrase inhibitors

Advanced renal failure (GFR < 20 ml/min)	Impairment of H^+ ion secretion
	  Renal insufficiency (GFR > 20 ml/min)
	  Distal RTA
	    Classic (type 1 RTA)
	    Aldosterone deficiency or resistance
	      (type 4 RTA)

Massive rhabdomyolysis	Miscellaneous
	  Parenteral hyperalimentation
	  Addition of HCl or its congeners
	  Recovery from ketoacidosis
	  Dilutional acidosis

mEq/L) are somewhat nonspecific with an excess unmeasured anion identified in only 30%. Metabolic acidosis may not be present in these mild situations; hyperproteinemia and hyperphosphatemia are thought to be contributory factors. However, when the AG is more than 20 mEq/L, metabolic acidosis is almost always present. Increased endogenous acid production is a frequent cause of a high AG acidosis with the most common causes being ketoacidosis and lactic acidosis.

Normal Anion Gap (Hyperchloremic)

On the other hand, normal AG metabolic acidosis results from either the addition of HCl to the body or the loss of bicarbonate from the gastrointestinal tract or the kidney. If HCl is added to the body, extracellular HCO_3^- is replaced by Cl^-; thus, there is no change in the anion gap since the sum ($[Cl^-] + HCO_3^-]$) remains constant. In gastrointestinal and renal losses of bicarbonate, the kidney retains Cl^- in place of the wasted HCO_3^-.

The major causes of metabolic acidosis with a normal anion gap (Table 5-1) are the result of bicarbonate losses from the gastrointestinal tract or the urine.

GENERAL READINGS

Arruda JAL, Kurtzman NA: Mechanisms and classification of deranged distal urinary acidification. Am J Physiol 239:F515, 1980

Emmett M, Narins RG: Clinical use of the anion gap. Medicine 56:38, 1977

Gabow PA: Disorders associated with an altered anion gap. Kidney Int 27:472, 1985

Halperin ML, Jungas RL: Metabolic production and renal disposal of hydrogen ions. Kidney Int 24:709, 1983

Kurtzman NA: Renal tubular acidosis: a constellation of syndromes. Hosp Practice 22:173, 1987

CASE STUDY 1

Metabolic Acidosis Secondary to Diabetic Ketoacidosis

Miss Zucchero, a 28-year-old woman with a 15-year history of diabetes mellitus, was brought to the hospital in a coma. She was afebrile, but breathing rapidly and deeply. Her blood pressure was 120/70, and her pulse 90/min and regular with orthostatic changes in both BP and pulse. There were no other neurologic findings. Apart from diabetic retinopathy, the remainder of her physical examination was normal.

LABORATORY DATA

Glucose 500 mg/dL	BUN 20 mg/dL
Serum ketones not done	Creatinine 1.3 mg/dL
Na^+ 133 mEq/L	Arterial blood pH 7.08
K^+ 4.0 mEq/L	$PaCO_2$ 14 mmHg
Cl^- 96 mEq/L	PaO_2 98 mmHg
HCO_3^- 4 mmol/L	

Question 1. What are the clues in the history and physical examination that lead to the diagnosis of the underlying disorder?

Question 2. What is the etiology of the acid-base disturbance?

Question 3. How would you diagnose the acid-base disturbance?

Question 4. What other conditions are associated with ketoacidosis?

Question 5. What is the appropriate therapy?

1. What are the clues in the history and physical examination that lead to the diagnosis of the underlying disorder?

The low serum bicarbonate raises the suspicion that the patient has a metabolic acidosis. When faced with a patient with suspected metabolic acidosis, it is good practice to follow a systematic approach as shown in Figure 5-3. One should first obtain measurements of blood pH and PaCO$_2$, not only to verify the clinical impression but also to assess the adequacy of the secondary physiologic responses. A low pH associated with low serum HCO$_3^-$ concentration confirms the diagnosis of metabolic acidosis. An elevated pH points to the diagnosis of respiratory alkalosis in which the primary disturbance is a lowered PaCO$_2$; the renal compensation that follows in this setting consists of increasing renal bicarbonate excretion with a resultant decrease in plasma bicarbonate. If on the other hand the pH is normal, one should suspect a mixed acid-base disorder. In metabolic acidosis, respiratory compensation lowers PaCO$_2$. The appropriateness of the respiratory compensation can be calculated by applying the Winters' formula.

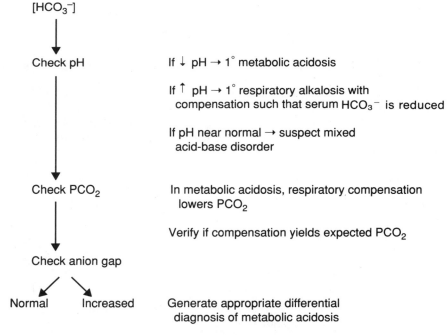

Fig. 5-3. Approach to the patient with metabolic acidosis.

In this case, the associated low arterial blood pH verifies that her primary acid-base disturbance is metabolic acidosis. The expected arterial $PaCO_2$ according to the Winters' formula is $(1.5 \times 4) + 8 = 14$ mmHg. The measured arterial $PaCO_2$ corresponds to the expected value indicating that the patient has an appropriate respiratory compensation. Calculation of the AG indicates that the disturbance is a high AG metabolic acidosis (AG $= 133 - (96 + 4) = 33$ mEq/L).

2. What is the etiology of the acid-base disturbance?

The etiology of the high anion gap metabolic acidosis is most likely secondary to diabetic ketoacidosis. Diabetic ketoacidosis appears to require insulin deficiency coupled with a relative or absolute increase in glucagon secretion. It is often caused by cessation of insulin intake, but may result from physical or emotional stress despite continued insulin therapy. The lack of insulin increases lipolysis and free fatty acid delivery to the liver while the excess of glucagon indirectly increases fatty acyl CoA entry into the hepatic mitochondria, where it can be converted into ketones. The short-chain fatty ketoacid, acetoacetic acid, and β-hydroxybutyrate, are the major acids produced in uncontrolled diabetes. These acids dissociate rapidly into H^+ and ketoanions resulting in metabolic acidosis with an increased anion gap. However, in this case, hypotension may also result in impaired tissue oxygenation, which is an ideal setting for the development of lactic acidosis.

3. How would you diagnose the acid-base disturbance?

The diagnosis of ketoacidosis is usually made using the nitroprusside reaction (Acetest) in the serum or urine. This test can yield false negative results, however, since it will identify acetone and acetoacetate but not β-hydroxybutyrate, which usually constitutes about two-thirds of the plasma ketoanions. Higher levels of β-hydroxybutyrate (and, therefore, a possible negative test) may be found in patients with concurrent lactic acidosis. An indirect way to get around this problem is by adding a few drops of hydrogen peroxide to a urine specimen resulting in the generation of detectable acetoacetate. Whether lactic acidosis is also present in the setting of ketoacidosis requires confirmation by measurements of blood lactate level.

4. What other conditions are associated with ketoacidosis?

Alcoholic ketoacidosis can occur after a period of heavy alcohol use. In addition to decreased carbohydrate intake, alcohol contributes to ketone formation by promoting the release of free fatty acids from adipose tissue. Since a preponderance of β-hydroxybutyric acid is usually seen, the Acetest in the serum or the urine may be negative, and the diagnosis is usually made by exclusion. In some cases, a concomitant lactic acidosis is present, which also gives a negative nitroprusside reaction test. Starvation is also associated with an increased breakdown of fatty acids and a mild ketosis is frequently seen. The plasma HCO_3^- concentration, however, does not decrease to less than 18 mmol/L.

5. What is the appropriate therapy?

Insulin is the specific therapy to correct the acidosis of diabetic ketoacidosis. Administration of fluids and electrolyte-replacement therapy that includes potassium, phosphate, and occasionally magnesium, are also essential. Bicarbonate administration is not indicated in most patients with ketoacidosis since metabolism of the ketoacid anions results in the regeneration of bicarbonate and spontaneous correction of the acidosis. Small amounts of sodium bicarbonate may be beneficial, however, when severe acidemia exists (pH < 7.1); it can be given to raise the pH to 7.20.

In this case, the amount of bicarbonate is roughly estimated by: (desired $[HCO_3^-]$ − measured $[HCO_3^-]$) × 50% body weight (kg); e.g., (12 mmol/L–4 mmol/L) × 0.5 × 70 = 280 mmol of $NaHCO_3$. This is only a rough estimate since the bicarbonate space depends on the level of HCO_3^- concentration (the lower the concentration, the bigger the space), and frequent arterial blood gases should be obtained to prevent overshooting the desired pH.

CASE STUDY 2

Metabolic Acidosis Secondary to Shock-Induced Lactic Acidosis

Mr. Sangue, a 45-year-old man weighing 70 kg, had acute gastrointestinal bleeding, followed by hypotension and confusion. He was noted to have labored breathing.

LABORATORY DATA

Glucose 126 mg/dL	BUN 90 mg/dL
Na^+ 140 mEq/L	Creatinine 1.2 mg/dL
K^+ 4.2 mEq/L	Arterial blood pH 6.97
Cl^- 104 mEq/L	$PaCO_2$ 12 mmHg
HCO_3^- 3 mEq/L	PaO_2 96 mmHg

Question 1. Considering the clinical setting, what is the most likely cause?
Question 2. What is the acid-base disturbance?
Question 3. What mechanism could be responsible for the acid-base disturbance?
Question 4. What laboratory test would help you make the diagnosis?
Question 5. What is the appropriate therapy?

---

1. Considering the clinical setting, what is the most likely cause?

Lactic acidosis is the most likely cause of the metabolic acidosis in this case. It is actually the most common cause of metabolic acidosis in hospitalized patients. Both overproduction and decreased metabolic conversion of lactate appear to be operative in most patients with lactic acidosis. Lactate is synthesized reversibly from pyruvate in a reaction catalyzed by lactate dehydrogenase (LDH): H-pyruvate + NADH → H-lactate + NAD. The normal rate of lactate production is 15 to 20 mEq/kg/day, most of which occurs via the glycolytic pathway that converts glucose into pyruvate. Anaerobic conditions, however, favor the conversion of pyruvate into lactate.

2. What is the acid-base disturbance?

The patient has metabolic acidosis as his primary acid-base disturbance as evidenced by a low serum bicarbonate concentration and an associated low arterial blood pH. The AG is high (33 mEq/L) and the measured arterial $PaCO_2$ (12 mmHg) corresponds to the expected value obtained by Winters' formula (12.5 mmHg) indicating that the patient has an appropriate respiratory compensation.

3. What mechanism could be responsible for the acid-base disturbance?

Lactic acidosis is usually caused by impaired tissue oxygenation (type A) due to shock, sepsis, or hypoxemia. Patients will have a low systemic blood pressure; cool, clammy extremities; oligoanuria; and impaired mental status. However, there is another type of lactic acidosis (type B) where findings of systemic hypoperfusion are not apparent and which is usually due to a toxin-induced impairment of cellular metabolism. With malignancy, for example, anaerobic metabolism by clusters of tumor cells in the liver may play a role. Table 5-2 lists some of the common causes of lactic acidosis. In comparison to patients with mineral acid-induced acidemia (as with renal failure or diarrhea), the plasma potassium does not rise in organic acidoses (such as lactic acidosis or ketoacidosis). When hyperkalemia occurs in the setting of organic acidoses, it is usually due to the cellular release of potassium due to ischemic cell breakdown.

4. What laboratory tests would help you make the diagnosis?

The history of hypotension that is associated with impaired tissue oxygenation is an ideal setting for the development of lactic acidosis. However, one should exclude other causes of metabolic acidosis associated with an increased anion gap. A plasma lactate level can help the diagnosis. The normal value for lactate ranges from 0.3 to 1.3 mmol/L. The liver and, to a lesser extent, the kidney are the major organs that remove lactate from the circulation. In both organs, lactate is converted back to pyruvate and in turn to glucose. Significant lactic acidosis (lactate >5 mmol/L) develops only when lactate production exceeds hepatic metabolism or renal excretion.

Table 5-2. Classification of Lactic Acidosis

Type A	Type B
Increased oxygen demand	Acquired
Generalized convulsions	Uncontrolled diabetes mellitus
Severe exercise	Certain malignancies
Hypothermic shivering	Hypoglycemia
	D-Lactic acidosis
Reduced oxygen delivery	
Shock	Toxins
Low cardiac output	Ethanol
Cardiac arrest	Methanbol
Sepsis	Ethylene glycol
Severe hypoxemia	Phenformin
Carbon monoxide poisoning	Salicylates
Cyanide intoxication	
	Pheochromocytoma
	Hepatic failure
	Acute respiratory alkalosis
	Congenital (e.g., glycogen storage disease, type 1)

5. What is the appropriate therapy?

Correction of the underlying disorder is the primary therapy for lactic acidosis. Restoration of adequate oxygenation and perfusion of tissues, and replacement of electrolyte deficits constitute the necessary supportive therapy.

The use of alkali therapy in the treatment of lactic acidosis is controversial. The potential benefit of bicarbonate therapy is maintenance of normal cardiovascular homeostasis. This potential benefit must be weighted against the possible deleterious effects, such as volume overload, hyperosmolarity (44.6 mmol $NaHCO_3$ in 50 ml ampule), and overshoot alkalosis due to infused bicarbonate and restoration of tissue perfusion. The last problem results from the regeneration of bicarbonate when excess lactate is metabolized. In addition to these risks, experimental studies suggest that bicarbonate therapy may be ineffective due to an associated increase in lactate production. Bicarbonate therapy leads to a local increase in PCO_2 which can exacerbate the intracellular acidosis, since CO_2 rapidly enters the cell. This can lead to decreased lactate use in hepatic cells.

There are two possible future alternatives to bicarbonate therapy. One is the administration of dichloracetate (DCA) which increases the oxidation of pyruvate to acetylCoA. It has shown promise experimentally and in some patients with lactic acidosis, but it does not improve prognosis. The second alternative is the use of sodium carbonate (Na_2CO_3) as a source of alkali. Buffering of excess H^+ ions in this setting will lead to the generation of bicarbonate, not CO_2 that can worsen intracellular acidosis.

CASE STUDY 3

Metabolic Acidosis Secondary to Toxin-Associated Lactic Acidosis

Mr. Birra, a 42-year-old alcoholic man, was brought to the hospital in a coma. Physical examination revealed a blood pressure of 130/80 and a respiratory rate of 24/minute. Mild hepatosplenomegaly was present, but there was no edema or jaundice. There were no focal neurologic signs. Fundoscopic examination was inadequate.

LABORATORY DATA

BUN 30 mg/dl	Creatinine 1.5 mg/dL
Glucose 90 mg/dL	Blood ketones trace positive
Na^+ 140 mEq/L	Arterial pH 7.05
K^+ 5.5 mEq/L	$PaCO_2$ 16 mmHg
Cl^- 105 mEq/L	PaO_2 88 mmHg
HCO_3^- 6 mmol/L	Serum osmolality 340 mOsm/kg

Question 1. What is the acid-base disturbance?
Question 2. What may cause this acid-base disturbance in alcoholics?
Question 3. What additional physical or laboratory findings would help with the differential diagnosis of the acid-base disturbance?

Question 4. How does the serum osmolality help with the diagnosis in this case?
Question 5. How would you treat this disturbance?

1. What is the acid-base disturbance?

The low serum bicarbonate in association with a low arterial blood pH indicates that the patient has metabolic acidosis as a primary cause of his acid-base disturbance. Calculation of the AG indicates that the disturbance is a high AG metabolic acidosis (AG = 29 mEq/L). The expected arterial $PaCO_2$ according to the Winters' formula is 14 ± 2 mmHg. The measured arterial $PaCO_2$ corresponds to the expected value indicating that there is appropriate respiratory compensation.

2. What may cause this acid-base disturbance in alcoholics?

The differential diagnosis should essentially include all of the causes of a high anion gap metabolic acidosis. Of course specific lab data rule out some etiologies; e.g., a creatinine level of 1.5 eliminates severe renal failure as a cause. Particular concerns in the alcoholic patient are alcoholic ketoacidosis and lactic acidosis secondary to bacterial sepsis or toxin ingestion. Overdosage with several potential toxins may result in a severe high AG metabolic acidosis caused by the overproduction of various endogenous acids. Such potential poisons include salicylates, methanol, ethylene glycol (antifreeze) and, very rarely, paraldehyde. A variety of other agents may cause metabolic acidosis with an increased anion gap. Table 5-3 shows characteristic features associated with certain intoxications.

Ingestion of large amounts of salicylates may lead to serious metabolic and acid-base abnormalities. Salicylates have a central ventilation-stimulating effect that leads to hyperventilation, hypocapnia, and respiratory alkalosis. Metabolic acidosis with an increased anion gap also results from the accumulation of salicylic acid and other organic acid intermediates. A mixed respiratory alkalosis and metabolic acidosis with an increased anion gap is seen in over 50% of adults with salicylate intoxication. The diagnosis of salicylism in the adult is suggested by a history of aspirin ingestion, nausea and tinnitus, and by the presence of unexplained hyperventilation, noncardiogenic pulmonary edema, an elevated prothrombin time, and a positive urine ferric chloride test.

Table 5-3. Characteristic Features of Poisoning with Toxins Causing High Anion Gap Metabolic Acidosis

Etiology	Major Circulating Anions	Characteristic Features
Methanol	Formate	Increased osmolal gap; hyperemic optic disk with retinal sheen.
Ethylene glycol	Glycolate, lactate	Increased osmolal gap; acute renal failure; urinary oxalate crystals; hypocalcemia. Coma and pulmonary edema can occur in severe cases.
Salicylates	Variety of organic acids; salicylate	Concomitant respiratory alkalosis; tinnitus.
Toluene	?Hippurate	Can also cause distal renal tubular acidosis.
Paraldehyde	?Acetate	Rare; previous cases may have misdiagnosed patients with alcoholic ketoacidosis.

A high salicylate blood level is diagnostic, but correlates poorly with symptoms. It is the non-ionized acid form, rather than the salicylate ion itself, that enters the brain. Acidemia increases the amount of non-ionized acid and thus worsens the neurologic symptoms. Treatment of salicylate intoxication should be directed at preventing or correcting acidemia. Therapy includes intravenous administration of bicarbonate in order to alkalinize the urine (urine pH >7.0), which will enhance the renal clearance of salicylate.

Methanol and ethylene glycol intoxication are among the few causes of metabolic acidosis with anion gaps greater than 50 mEq/L. Patients with methanol intoxication often complain of abdominal pain, vomiting, headache, and visual disturbances. Retinitis leading to blindness develops about 12 to 18 hours after a toxic dose of methanol, and is secondary to the accumulation of the toxic metabolite, formic acid, that is produced by the oxidation of methyl alcohol by alcohol dehydrogenase. Ethanol infusion delays the oxidation of methyl alcohol, thereby reducing the accumulation of toxic metabolites. Ethylene glycol ingestion can lead to CNS disturbances, cardiovascular collapse, respiratory failure, and renal failure. The acidosis is due to the accumulation of glycolic acid. Large amounts of oxalate crystals may be seen in the urine and are diagnostic. Treatment with ethanol also retards the metabolism of ethylene glycol, and allows time for renal excretion. A clue to the diagnosis of intoxication by methanol or ethylene glycol is an increase in the osmolal gap in addition to the elevated anion gap. It should be noted that intoxication with ethanol results in an elevation of the osmolal gap without a corresponding increase in the anion gap (unless alcoholic ketoacidosis or lactic acidosis are also present). The normal osmolal gap (obtained by subtracting the calculated from the measured plasma osmolality) is less than 10, and consists mainly of calcium, lipids, and proteins. The Posm can be calculated from the following formula: Posm (calculated) $= 2[Na^+] + [glucose]/18 + BUN/2.8$. An osmolal gap, i.e., a difference of greater than 10 mOsm between the measured and the calculated osmolality, is consistent with the ingestion of an osmotically active agent such as methanol, ethylene glycol, or ethanol. Its increase can also be a feature of acute renal failure.

3. What additional physical or laboratory findings would help with the differential diagnosis of the acid-base disturbance?

On fundoscopic examination, hyperemic discs would be seen in a patient who has ingested methanol. Calcium oxalate crystals would be seen in the urine of a patient who has ingested ethylene glycol. Obtaining a blood-alcohol level would certainly be beneficial. A positive serum ketone level would be helpful in the evaluation of alcoholic ketoacidosis. If a severe lactic acidosis is present, however, any ketones present may be in the form of β-hydroxybutyrate, which is not detected by the ketone assay in the laboratory. Very low glucose levels may be seen in alcoholic ketoacidosis as well.

4. How does the serum osmolality help with the diagnosis in this case?

The osmolal gap in this problem is clearly greater than 10 since the measured osmolality is 340 while the calculated osmolality is: $2[Na^+] + glucose/18 + BUN/2.8 = 2 \times 140 + 90/18 + 30/2.8 = 296$ mOsm. This is consistent with the ingestion of an osmotically active agent, such as methanol or ethylene glycol. Note that ethanol ingestion can also lead to a high osmolal gap without an increase of the anion gap unless there is an associated alcoholic ketoacidosis or lactic acidosis.

5. How would you treat this disturbance?

Treatment consists of vigorous volume replacement, administration of glucose, and repletion of potassium, magnesium, and phosphorous deficits. It is also important to observe for early alcohol-related signs and symptoms of withdrawal.

CASE STUDY 4

Metabolic Acidosis Secondary to Chronic Renal Failure

Mr. Bjorn Wittit, a 25-year-old man, has been followed for progressive renal failure due to vesico-ureteral reflux and recurrent urinary tract infections for the past 20 years. Apart from mild hypertension controlled with a low sodium diet (BP 126/82), his physical examination was entirely normal.

LABORATORY DATA		
5 years ago	1 month ago	Today
BUN 30 mg/dL	BUN 72 mg/dL	BUN 80 mg/dL
Na^+ 142 mEq/L	Na^+ 144 mEq/L	Na^+ 139 mEq/L
K^+ 4.8 mEq/L	K^+ 5.2 mEq/L	K^+ 5.6 mEq/L
Cl^- 108 mEq/L	Cl^- 107 mEq/L	Cl^- 105 mEq/L
HCO_3^- 22 mmol/L	HCO_3^- 16 mmol/L	HCO_3^- 14 mmol/L

Question 1. What acid-base disturbance is most likely at each time?
Question 2. What is the pathogenesis of metabolic acidosis in this condition?
Question 3. Why is the anion gap changing?
Question 4. Assuming that the patient has been on a normal diet, what would be appropriate therapy to correct his acid-base disturbance?
Question 5. How would your daily therapy be influenced by a protein-restricted diet?
Question 6. How would your therapy be influenced if the urinary pH was never less than 7.0 (even when no infection is present)?

---

1. What acid-base disturbance is likely at each time?

The acid-base disturbance seen in this patient is a metabolic acidosis that has worsened over time. This is most likely related in this case to worsening renal failure. Calculation of the AG reveals that the patient had a normal AG of 12 mEq/L early in his disease course. However, as his renal disease progressed, the worsening of the metabolic acidosis was accompanied by an increase in AG, to its present level of 20 mEq/L.

2. What is the pathogenesis of metabolic acidosis in this condition?

In renal insufficiency, metabolic acidosis is due to the inability of the kidney to excrete all of the daily H^+ load. This is mostly the result of a decline in total ammonium excretion resulting from a decrease in the renal mass. Total ammonium excretion begins to fall when the GFR is less than 40 to 50 mL/min. Decreased titrable acidity (primarily as phosphate) and reduced

HCO_3^- reabsorption also contribute, although to a much lesser extent, to the decline in net acid excretion.

As the patient approaches end-stage renal failure, the plasma HCO_3^- concentration usually falls and then stabilizes around 12 to 20 mEq/L. Although H^+ ions continue to be retained, a further reduction in plasma HCO_3^- concentration is prevented by buffering of the excess acid by bone. This results in a relative increase in calcium release from the bone and can be reversed by correction of the acidemia. A plasma HCO_3^- concentration below 10 to 12 mEq/L is usually due to a superimposed metabolic acidosis.

3. Why is the anion gap changing?

The metabolic acidosis of renal failure can be characterized by either a normal or elevated anion gap (or both). The pathogenesis of the metabolic acidosis in renal failure (irrespective of the fate of the AG) is always due to the titration of HCO_3^- by the retained H^+. Whether the AG is elevated depends on whether the anions (sulfates and phosphates) that accompany the retained H^+ are excreted in the urine. These anions depend on filtration for their excretion. In severe renal failure (GFR <15 mL/min), there is a decrease in filtration and retention of these anions, while in mild to moderate renal failure (GFR 15–40 mL/min) these anions are freely excreted and do not accumulate.

4. Assuming that the patient has been on a normal diet, what would be appropriate therapy to correct his acid-base disturbance?

The limited fall in the plasma HCO_3^- concentration and the respiratory compensation usually maintain the arterial pH near 7.30. Appropriate therapy to correct the metabolic acidosis of renal failure would consist of oral bicarbonate (or its equivalent) replacement, usually to maintain the serum bicarbonate level greater than 15 to 18 mmol/L. Citrate as a bicarbonate equivalent should be avoided in patients who are also taking aluminum-containing phosphate binders, as it may increase aluminum absorption from the gut. Attention should be given to preventing a rise in the pH in the presence of hypocalcemia, as it can precipitate tetany and the associated Na^+ load can increase the tendency toward volume expansion.

To preserve the serum bicarbonate level within the normal range, the patient will require an amount of bicarbonate equal to the amount of nonvolatile acid produced daily. Since the average meat-eating individual produces approximately 1 mEq/kg body weight of nonvolatile acid per day, replacement therapy would consist of 70 mEq of bicarbonate per day in a 70 kg patient. Early treatment of mild metabolic acidosis in renal failure has also been advocated in order to prevent or delay the development of osteopenia, and to minimize the loss of lean body mass and muscle weakness.

5. How would your daily therapy be influenced by a protein-restricted diet?

Since most nonvolatile acids come from the metabolism of animal proteins, protein restriction is usually associated with less nonvolatile acid production. Therefore, less bicarbonate replacement therapy would be needed. It is important also to restrict phosphorus intake to prevent or minimize hyperparathyroidism. In addition, phosphate binders can be used. Nonaluminum phosphate binders are preferred to avoid the problem of aluminum toxicity.

6. How would your therapy be influenced if the urinary pH was never less than 7.0 (even when no infection is present)?

Since patients with renal failure retain the ability to lower the urine pH to between 4.5 and 5.5 even at low levels of GFR, a relatively alkaline urine (pH 7.0) indicates that the kidneys are losing bicarbonate, in addition to their inability to excrete nonvolatile acids. This means that more bicarbonate replacement therapy would be needed.

CASE STUDY 5

Metabolic Acidosis Secondary to Diarrhea

Miss Ginny King, a 78-year-old woman, was admitted to the hospital with episodic diarrhea and weight loss for 3 months. Physical examination revealed only evidence of volume depletion. During the first week in the hospital the patient was observed to have 8 to 10 watery bowel movements/day and lost 5 lbs from her admission weight despite medication to control her diarrhea.

LABORATORY DATA

Admission	After 1 week	
BUN 18 mg/dL	BUN 28 mg/dL	Arterial blood: pH 7.24
Na^+ 138 mEq/L	Na^+ 135 mEq/L	$PaCO_2$ 27 mmHg
K^+ 3.9 mEq/L	K^+ 3.0 mEq/L	PaO_2 100 mmHg
Cl^- 100 mEq/L	Cl^- 110 mEq/L	
HCO_3^- 27 mmol/L	HCO_3^- 13 mmol/L	

Question 1. What is the acid-base disturbance after 1 week?
Question 2. What is the cause of the acid-base disturbance?
Question 3. What other gastrointestinal disturbances can cause an acidosis?
Question 4. What is the cause of the fall in serum K^+ concentration?
Question 5. Assuming no further diarrhea, what would be appropriate treatment?

---

1. What is the acid-base disturbance after 1 week?

The lower serum bicarbonate in association with a low arterial blood pH indicates that the patient has metabolic acidosis as a primary cause of her acid-base disturbance. Calculation of the AG indicates that the disturbance is a normal AG metabolic acidosis (AG = 12 mEq/L). The expected arterial $PaCO_2$ according to the Winters' formula is 27.5 ± 2 mmHg. The measured arterial $PaCO_2$ corresponds to the expected value, which indicates that appropriate respiratory compensation is present.

2. What is the cause of the acid-base disturbance?

The most obvious cause for this disturbance is profuse diarrhea. Diarrhea is by far the most common cause of hyperchloremic metabolic acidosis and should always be considered first in the differential diagnosis of hyperchloremic metabolic acidosis. The concentration of HCO_3^- in diarrheal fluid is usually greater than in plasma, leading to significant bicarbonate losses. The patient has been losing both bicarbonate and organic salts like acetate and pyruvate in her stools, which are potential sources of bicarbonate in the body.

3. What other gastrointestinal disturbances can cause an acidosis?

Secretions from the small bowel (600–700 mL/day), biliary system (>1 L/day), and pancreas (>2 L/day) are rich in HCO_3^- and poor in Cl^-. As a result, tube drainage or external fistulas from these sites will lead to a normal AG metabolic acidosis. Large amounts of bicarbonate losses in the urine also occur in pancreatic transplantation with anastomosis of the pancreatic duct into the urinary bladder.

Metabolic acidosis commonly occurs with ureterosigmoidostomy (ureters drained into the sigmoid colon after removal of the bladder). In this setting, during the period of retention of the urine in the colon, passive chloride and H_2O reabsorption occurs; there is also active HCO_3^- secretion, which will lead to a net loss of HCO_3^- and the development of hyperchloremic metabolic acidosis. An obstructed ileal loop conduit may give rise to the same problem. In both instances, the urine is initially normal, but prolonged exposure to bowel mucosa leads to external losses of HCO_3^-.

Anion exchange resins such as cholestyramine have some affinity for HCO_3^- and may exchange chloride for HCO_3^- across the bowel mucosa. Patients with compromised renal function may be unable to generate new HCO_3^- and thus excrete the absorbed chloride, leading to a hyperchloremic metabolic acidosis.

If large amounts of $CaCl_2$ or $MgCl_2$ are taken by mouth, the unabsorbed Ca or Mg reacts with HCO_3^-, which has been exchanged across the gut mucosa for chloride, to form an insoluble carbonate salt. This will lead to a fall in plasma HCO_3^- and a rise in plasma chloride.

4. What is the cause of the fall in serum K^+ concentration?

Prominent stool K losses occur in diarrheic states, and K depletion develops commonly. Although K is lost in the diarrhea, the greatest loss of K occurs in the urine because of the increased aldosterone levels stimulated by the diarrhea-induced volume contraction.

5. Assuming no further diarrhea, what would be appropriate treatment?

Assuming on further diarrhea, the patient will need volume replacement in the range of several liters of isotonic saline. Potassium replacement would be needed as well, and based on a serum K^+ level of 3.0 mEq/L, the K^+ deficit may be as high as 200 mEq. At this point, no bicarbonate therapy would be needed. The patient would essentially replete her bicarbonate concentration stores through renal regeneration at the distal tubule. If the bicarbonate concentration were lower (e.g., <11 mmol/L), then generally the patient should receive oral bicarbonate replacement therapy or its equivalent (e.g., sodium citrate).

CASE STUDY 6

Metabolic Acidosis Secondary to Renal Tubular Acidosis

Mr. Pietra, a 23-year-old man with a history of calcium oxalate stone, presented to the hospital after having just passed another radio-opaque stone. He denied any history of drug ingestion or gastrointestinal disorder, but does have a family history of stone disease. Physical examination is entirely normal.

LABORATORY DATA

BUN 15 mg/dL	Creatinine 1.0 mg/dL
Na^+ 140 mEq/L	Calcium 9.2 mg/dL
K^+ 3.0 mEq/L	Phosphorous 4.0 mg/dL
Cl^- 115 mEq/L	Uric acid 4.0 mg/dL
HCO_3^- 15 mmol/L	Total protein 6.0 g/dL
Arterial blood pH 7.35	(Albumin/Globulin normal)

Urinalysis: Negative except for a pH of 7.2

Question 1. What is the acid-base disturbance most likely to be?
Question 2. Given the clinical setting, what is the most likely diagnosis?
Question 3. What is the pathophysiologic basis for this disorder?
Question 4. How would you treat this disorder?

---

1. What is the acid-base disturbance most likely to be?

The patient has a metabolic acidosis based on the low serum bicarbonate and the associated low arterial blood pH. Calculation of the anion gap indicates that the disturbance is a normal AG metabolic acidosis. $(AG = 140 - (115 + 15) = 10$ mEq/L).

2. Given the clinical setting, what is the most likely diagnosis?

In the absence of infection or volume depletion, the differential diagnosis of a normal AG with a high urine pH consists of type 1 and 2 RTA. Renal tubular acidosis (RTA) refers to a group of disorders characterized by defective H^+ secretion by the kidney or by the renal loss of bicarbonate. There are two major types of RTA, distal, or Type 1, RTA and proximal, or Type 2, RTA, named for the renal tubular segments where the presumed defect exists. Both conditions lead to a hyperchloremic metabolic acidosis. The history of recurrent nephrolithiasis suggests the diagnosis of type 1 RTA. Type 1 RTA is frequently associated with renal calculi and nephrocalcinosis. Reduced excretion of citrate, a urinary inhibitor of calcium stone formation, is the principal cause for nephrolithiasis in distal RTA.

3. What is the pathophysiologic basis for this disorder?

Distal RTA is a disorder in which the collecting duct fails to maximally acidify the urine. Normally, the urine pH can be lowered to 4.5 to 5.0 in the collecting tubules in the presence of an acid load. In comparison, patients with distal RTA cannot lower the urine pH below 5.3, even with severe acidemia. This results in an inability to excrete the dietary acid load and the net effect is a progressive metabolic acidosis, with a plasma bicarbonate that may fall below 10 mEq/L if untreated.

The classic feature of type 1 RTA is the presence of a normal anion gap metabolic acidosis with a urine pH that is persistently above 5.3. In addition to this defect in acid-base balance, K homeostasis is also frequently abnormal in this disorder. In most cases, hypokalemia is observed because, since net H^+ excretion is impaired, more Na must be reabsorbed in the cortical collecting tubule in exchange for K to maintain electroneutrality. However, hyperkalemia is also observed in cases of type 1 RTA due to urinary tract obstruction and sickle cell nephropathy, where the primary abnormality is a limitation in sodium reabsorption. Some of the entities associated with type 1 RTA are listed in Table 5-4. In children, growth failure or bone disease

Table 5-4. Causes of Renal Tubular Acidosis (RTA)

Distal RTA	Proximal RTA
Primary	Hereditary
Idiopathic or sporadic	Cystinosis
Genetic	Tyrosinemia
Familial	Wilson's disease
Marfan's syndrome	Glycogen storage disease, type I
Wilson's disease	Pyruvate carboxylase deficiency
Ehler-Danlos syndrome	Galactosemia
Disorders of calcium metabolism with nephrocalcinosis	Acquired disorders
Idiopathic hypercalciuria	Multiple myeloma
Hypervitaminosis D	Vitamin D deficiency
Chronic hyperparathyroidism	Nephrotic syndrome
Hypergammaglobulinemic states	Amyloidosis
Amyloidosis	Renal transplant rejection
Multiple myeloma	Sjögren's syndrome
Cryoglobulinemia	Toxins and drugs
Drugs and toxins	Lead
Amphotericin B	Cadmium
Lithium carbonate	Mercury
Toluene	Uranium
Autoimmune diseases	Copper (Wilson's disease)
Sjögren syndrome	Acetazolamide
Thyroiditis	Outdated tetracycline
Chronic active hepatitis	Streptozotocin
Primary biliary cirrhosis	
Miscellaneous	
Cirrhosis	
Medullary sponge kidney	
Associated with hyperkalemia	
Urinary tract obstruction	
Sickle cell anemia	
Systemic lupus erythematosus	
Renal transplant rejection	

are also observed. Autoimmune diseases like Sjögren syndrome are the major causes of this condition in adults, whereas hereditary RTA is most common in children.

Hypoaldosteronism or tubular resistance to the action of aldosterone is the most common cause of hyperkalemic distal RTA (often referred to as type IV distal RTA). Hypoaldosteronism is more commonly associated with hyporeninism, and occurs more frequently in older patients, particularly those with diabetes mellitus and mild to moderate renal failure. Tubular resistance to aldosterone action is commonly seen in partial obstruction of the urinary tract and in tubulo-interstitial nephritides. Aldosterone stimulates distal nephron H^+ and K secretion as well as Na reabsorption. Therefore, absent or reduced aldosterone production can manifest as hyperchloremic metabolic acidosis, hyperkalemia, and volume depletion. Metabolic acidosis in this setting is caused in part by decreased NH_3 production due to hyperkalemia and in part by decreased renal tubular H^+ secretion due to low aldosterone levels. Treatment of the hyperkalemia alone or use of mineralocorticoid replacement will ameliorate the acidosis. Mineralocorticoids must be used cautiously to avoid excessive Na^+ retention and hypertension.

4. How would you treat this disorder?

Treatment of distal RTA consists of providing sufficient alkali, from 1 to 3 mmol/kg/day, to maintain near normal acid-base status. This is equivalent to the daily net production of nonvolatile H^+. Alkali administration may reduce the renal losses of K, but some patients continue to require K supplements (e.g., K citrate, which also provides alkali).

CASE STUDY 7

Metabolic Acidosis in Fanconi's Syndrome

Joe Bambino, a 2-year-old boy, is admitted to the hospital because of failure to thrive.

LABORATORY DATA

Glucose 100 mg/dL	BUN 15 mg/dL
Na^+ 140 mEq/L	Calcium 9.2 mg/dL
K^+ 2.6 mEq/L	Phosphorous 1.8 mg/dL
Cl^- 115 mEq/L	Uric acid 1.2 mg/dL
HCO_3^- 15 mEq/L	Arterial pH 7.32

Urinalysis was significant for a pH = 7.0, positive urine glucose, 0–1 WBC/HPF, no bacteria. A urine culture was negative.

Question 1. What is the acid-base disturbance most likely to be?
Question 2. What condition does the boy most likely have?
Question 3. How can the diagnosis be confirmed?
Question 4. What would be adequate therapy?
Question 5. What other nonrenal disturbances can lead to a similar type of acidosis?

1. What is the acid-base disturbance most likely to be?

The patient has a metabolic acidosis based on the low serum bicarbonate and the associated low arterial blood pH. Calculation of the anion gap indicates that the disturbance is a normal AG metabolic acidosis. ($AG = 140 - (115 + 15) = 10$ mEq/L).

2. What condition does the boy most likely have?

The etiology of the normal AG metabolic acidosis is most likely secondary to type 2 (proximal) renal tubular acidosis. The blood phosphorus and uric acid levels are low and there is evidence of glucosuria, indicating that the patient has a Fanconi syndrome. With proximal RTA, the proximal tubular reclamation of HCO_3^-, which normally accounts for more than 90% of filtered bicarbonate, is defective. This results in bicarbonate diuresis, since the distal nephron has only a limited capacity to reclaim HCO_3^-. Maximal urine acidification can be achieved in proximal RTA when the plasma HCO_3^- concentration, and therefore the filtered HCO_3^- load, is reduced to a level at which the distal nephron can completely reclaim the amount of HCO_3^- delivered. The bicarbonaturia seen in proximal RTA induces renal losses of Na and K; therefore, volume depletion and hypokalemia also occur. In addition to HCO_3^-, glucose, phosphate, amino acids, and uric acid may also be inadequately reabsorbed in the proximal tubule of a patient with Fanconi syndrome. This results in systemic problems, including osteomalacia, malnutrition, and failure to thrive. However, in contrast to distal RTA, nephrocalconosis and nephrolithiasis are uncommon in proximal RTA since citrate excretion is not reduced. Some of the entities that have been associated with proximal RTA are listed in Table 5-4.

Acetazolamide inhibits renal tubular cellular and luminal brush border carbonic anhydrase. The inhibition of hydrolysis of intraluminal carbonic acid to CO_2 and H_2O will allow H^+ concentration to increase in the lumen, thus creating a gradient against H^+ secretion, and will retard reabsorption of HCO_3^-. As a result, more Na is reabsorbed with chloride than with HCO_3^- leading to a mild to moderate hyperchloremic metabolic acidosis.

3. How can the diagnosis be confirmed?

The diagnosis of RTA should be suspected in any patient with metabolic acidosis and a urine pH above 5.3. Urinary tract infection caused by a urea-splitting organism must first be excluded, because it can raise the urine pH by enhancing the generation of ammonia from urea. In addition, patients with other forms of metabolic acidosis (such as diarrhea) who are also severely volume depleted may have a reversible defect in urinary acidification. In this setting, volume depletion enhances proximal reabsorption of Na, thus limiting the amount of Na available for distal reabsorption and subsequent stimulation of H secretion. This may result in an inability to lower the urine pH below 5.3 that can be corrected with volume replacement. Thus, the diagnosis of RTA should not be made if the urine Na concentration is below 10 to 15 mEq/L.

In the absence of infection or volume depletion, the differential diagnosis of a normal anion gap metabolic acidosis with a high urine pH consists of type 1 and type 2 RTA. These disorders can be distinguished by infusing $NaHCO_3$ to raise the plasma bicarbonate concentration to around 20 to 22 mEq/L, and then measuring the urine pH and the fractional excretion of bicarbonate.

$$\text{Fractional excretion } HCO_3^- (\%) = \frac{\text{urine } [HCO_3^-] \times \text{plasma } [\text{creatinine}] \times 100}{\text{plasma } [HCO_3^-] \times \text{urine } [\text{creatinine}]} \qquad \text{(Eq. 5-8)}$$

The urine pH will be unchanged in type 1 RTA and the fractional excretion of bicarbonate will remain below 3% since bicarbonate reabsorption is not impaired in this condition. In comparison,

Table 5-5.   Characteristics of Types 1, 2, and 4 RTA

	Type I (Distal)	Type 2 (Proximal)	Type 4
Basic defect	Decreased distal acidification	Decreased proximal HCO_3^- reabsorption	Aldosterone deficiency or resistance
Urine pH	>5.3	Variable: >5.3 if above reabsorptive threshold: <5.3 if below	Usually <5.3
Plasma $[HCO_3^-]$ (untreated)	May be <10 mEq/L	>12 mEq/L	>15 mEq/L
Fractional excretion of bicarbonate when plasma $[HCO_3^-]$ >20 mEq/L	<3	>15–20%	<3%
Diagnosis	Response to $NaHCO_3$ or ammonium chloride	Response to $NaHCO_3$	Measure plasma aldosterone concentration
Plasma $[K^+]$	Usually reduced or normal; rarely elevated	Normal or reduced	Elevated
Therapeutic amount of $NaHCO_3$ required to normalize plasma $[HCO_3^-]$	1–3 mEq/kg/day	10–15 mEq/kg/day	1–3 mEq/kg/day, may require no alkali if correct hyperkalemia
Nonelectrolyte complictions	Nephrocalcinosis and renal stones Osteomalacia uncommon	Rickets in children Osteomalacia or ostopenia in adults Calculi rare unless taking carbonic anhydrase inhibitor	None

in type 2 RTA, raising the plasma bicarbonate concentration above the reabsorptive threshold of the proximal tubule will result in marked bicarbonate diuresis, with the urine pH rising above 7.0 and the fractional excretion of bicarbonate exceeding 10%.

There is an incomplete form of type 1 RTA in which the urine cannot be fully acidified, but the plasma bicarbonate and the pH remain normal. This condition can be diagnosed by giving an acid load like ammonium chloride in a dose of 0.1 g/kg. Maintenance of the urine pH above 5.3 is indicative of an underlying acidification defect.

One way to differentiate RTA from conditions that have a normal acidification (such as diarrhea) is to calculate the urine anion gap. The urine anion gap is helpful in estimating the amount of urinary ammonium (which is an unmeasured cation).

$$\text{Urine anion gap} = ([Na^+] + [K^+]) - [Cl^-] \qquad \text{(Eq. 5-9)}$$

When acidification is normal, as in most cases of diarrhea, there is a relatively large quantity of ammonium that is excreted with chloride. As a result, the urine anion gap has a negative value, since the chloride concentration exceeds that of Na plus K. In comparison, a positive value indicates impaired ammonium excretion and is suggestive of one of the forms of RTA.

Table 5-5 lists some of the important features of the different types of renal tubular acidoses.

4. What would be adequate therapy?

Treatment of RTA consists of providing sufficient alkali in order to maintain near normal acid-base status. In proximal RTA, large amounts of alkali (10 mmol/kg/day) may be needed. Large K supplements are also necessary, since urinary K loss increases with the increasing bicarbonaturia that occurs with alkali therapy.

5. What other nonrenal disturbances can lead to a similar type of acidosis?

The compounds HCl, NH_4Cl, lysine HCl, and arginine HCl all contain a quantity of HCl. When any of these are administered, the H^+ titrates HCO_3^-, which is replaced by chloride, leading to hyperchloremic metabolic acidosis with normal anion gap.

Amino acid infusates usually contain organic cations in excess of organic anions. The other accompanying anion in these infusates is usually chloride. Metabolism of these amino acid cations produces H^+, which is buffered by HCO_3^-. As chloride is retained, the result can be a hyperchloremic metabolic acidosis. Provision of sufficient organic anions in the form of acetate, lactate, or citrate often prevents the development of metabolic acidosis.

Rapid ECF expansion with fluids that do not contain HCO_3^- will lead to a temporary decrease in HCO_3^- concentration. This fall in bicarbonate concentration is small (<10%) and is rapidly corrected by the kidneys.

Hyperparathyroidism may cause a reduction in proximal renal tubular HCO_3^- reabsorption leading to bicarbonaturia and a condition that resembles proximal RTA. Increased PTH also causes phosphaturia and a combination of hyperchloremia and hypophosphatemia is a useful clue for the presence of hyperparathyroidism. In most cases of primary hyperparathyroidism with hypercalcemia and hypercalciuria, nephrocalcinosis and nephrolithiasis also develop. The common association of metabolic acidosis in this setting is due to distal RTA resulting from involvement of the collecting ducts with nephrocalcinosis.

FURTHER READINGS

Battle DC: Renal tubular acidosis. Med Clin North Am 67:859, 1983

Battle DC: Segmental characterization of defects in collecting tubule acidification. Kidney Int 30:546, 1986

Battle DC, Sehy JT, Roseman MK et al: Clinical physiologic spectrum of acquired distal renal tubular acidosis. Kidney Int 20:389, 1981

Bersin RM, Arieff AI: Improved hemodynamic function during hypoxia with Carbicarb, a new agent for the management of acidosis. Circulation 77:227, 1988

Cahill GR Jr: Ketosis. Kidney Int 20:416, 1983

Davis GR, Morawski SG, Santa Ana CA et al: Evaluation of chloride/bicarbonate exchange in the human colon in vivo. J Clin Invest 71:201, 1983

Duckett JW, Gazak JM: Complications of ureterosigmoidostomy. Urol Clin North Am 10:473, 1983

Foster DW, McGarry JD: The metabolic derangements and treatment of diabetic ketoacidosis. N Engl J Med 309:159, 1983

Fraley DS, Adler S, Bruns F et al: Metabolic acidosis after hyperalimentation with casein hydrolysate. Ann Intern Med 88:352, 1978

Frommer JP: Lactic acidosis. Med Clin North Am 67:815, 1983

Gabow PA: Ethylene glycol intoxication. Am J Kid Dis 11:277, 1988

Gabow PA, Anderson RJ, Potts DE et al: Acid-base disturbances in the salicylate-intoxicated adult. Arch Intern Med 138:1481, 1978

Glasser L, Sternglanz PD, Combie J et al: Serum osmolality and its applicability to drug overdose. Am J Clin Pathol 60:695, 1973

Kreisberg RA: Lactate homeostasis and lactic acidosis. Ann Intern Med 92:227, 1980

Miller PD, Heinig RE, Waterhouse C: Treatment of alcoholic acidosis. Arch Int Med 138:67, 1978

Oh MS, Carroll HJ, Goldstein DA et al: Hyperchloremic acidosis during the recovery phase of diabetic ketosis. Ann Intern Med 89:925, 1978

Palmisano J, Gruver C, Adams ND: Absence of anion gap metabolic acidosis in severe methanol poisoning: a case report and review of the literature. Am J Kid Dis 9:441, 1987

Perez GO, Oster JR, Rogers A: Acid-base disturbances in gastrointestinal disease. Dig Dis Sci 32:1033, 1987

Sklar AH, Linas SL: The osmolal gap in renal failure. Ann Intern Med 98:480, 1983

Stacpoole PW: Lactic acidosis: the case against bicarbonate therapy. Ann Intern Med 105:276, 1986

Stacpoole PW, Harman EM, Curry HS et al: Treatment of lactic acidosis with dichloroacetate. N Engl J Med 309:390, 1983

Stacpoole PW, Wright EC, Baumgartner TG et al: A controlled clinical trial of dichloroacetate for treatment of lactic acidosis in adults. N Engl J Med 327:1564, 1992

Wallia R, Greenberg A, Piraino B et al: Serum electrolyte patterns in end-stage renal disease. Am J Kid Dis 8:98, 1986

Warnock DG: Uremic acidosis. Kidney Int 34:278, 1988

6

Metabolic Alkalosis

Robert A. Gayner
Pedro C. Fernandez

BASIC CONCEPTS

Metabolic alkalosis is an acid-base disturbance originating from an excess in the body's bicarbonate content. The resulting increase in the bicarbonate concentration ($[HCO_3^-]$) of body fluids causes an elevation in the pH of those fluids, as predicted from the Henderson-Hasselbalch equation.

The HCO_3^-/CO^2 buffer system is in equilibrium with all other buffers in the body. The alkaline pH shift resulting from addition of HCO_3^- alters the balance of nonbicarbonate buffers and causes their acid moieties to dissociate:

$$AH \Leftrightarrow A^- + H^+ \qquad \text{(Eq. 6-1)}$$

Some of the added HCO_3^- is titrated by the H^+ to CO_2 and H_2O:

$$HCO_3^- + H^+ \Leftrightarrow H_2CO_3 \Leftrightarrow CO_2 + H_2O \qquad \text{(Eq. 6-2)}$$

Up to one-fifth of any HCO_3^- added to the body is dissipated by titration to CO_2 gas. The remaining 80% is directly responsible for the observed increase in the body's HCO_3^- content; its apparent volume of distribution is equal to 40% of body weight.

Ventilatory Response

In metabolic alkalosis, alkalinization of the blood and respiratory center milieu causes hypoventilation. For this reason the typical biochemical picture of metabolic alkalosis includes an elevated serum $[HCO_3^-]$ (i.e., the metabolic alkalosis proper), alkalemia and an elevation in the $PaCO_2$. The latter is often referred to as "compensatory," on the basis that an elevated $PaCO_2$ tends to normalize the pH when the $[HCO_3^-]$ is high.

THE ROLE OF EXTERNAL H$^+$ BALANCE

Normal H$^+$ Balance

Consumption of a Western diet results in the addition of 60 to 100 mEq of H$^+$ per day to body fluids as a result of the metabolic production of several inorganic and organic nonvolatile acids. This process would lead to the titration and progressive decline in the body content of bicarbonate and other buffer anions, were it not for the daily addition of an equimolar amount of base to body fluids. This addition of base is largely mediated through the disposal of H$^+$ into the exterior milieu.

Essentially all ionic interactions between body fluids and external milieu take place through the gastrointestinal and renal ion-transporting lining epithelia. Hydrogen ions (H$^+$) originating from dissociation of H$_2$O are secreted into the lumen across the apical cell membrane. Cell CO$_2$ is then hydroxylated to HCO$_3^-$, a reaction catalyzed by carbonic anhydrase (Fig. 6-1). The ensuing increase in cell [HCO$_3^-$] promotes HCO$_3^-$ exit across the basolateral cell membrane. A steady state is achieved and for each mEq of H$^+$ disposed off into the lumen 1 mEq of HCO$_3^-$ is added to the blood (Fig. 6-1).

The renal tubules, in addition to reabsorbing all the filtered HCO$_3^-$, secrete into the lumen an amount of H$^+$ equal to that generated by nonvolatile acids. This results in constancy of the body's HCO$_3^-$ content. The secreted H$^+$ is excreted in the final urine in the form of titratable acid (TA) and NH$_{4+}$ (Fig. 6-2).

The Generation of a Metabolic Alkalosis

A metabolic alkalosis is initiated whenever the rate of addition of HCO$_3^-$ to body fluids exceeds the rate of nonvolatile H$^+$ production. This situation occasionally occurs through provision of exogenous base, but it most often results from increased external losses of H$^+$ in the urine or via the gastrointestinal tract.

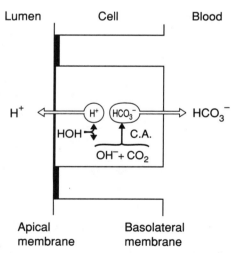

Fig. 6-1. Intracellular H$^+$ is secreted into the lumen across the apical cell membrane by specific H$^+$-translocating mechanisms located in that membrane. The (OH)$^-$ remaining in the cell is rapidly carboxylated to HCO$_3^-$ under the influence of cytoplasmic carbonic anhydrase (CA). Bicarbonate ion is then extruded from the cell across the basolateral cell membrane into the circulating blood. Both processes, apical H$^+$ secretion and basolateral HCO$_3^-$ extrusion, are inextricably linked to each other, so that secretion of 1 mEq of H$^+$ into the lumen results in the addition of 1 mEq of HCO$_3^-$ to the blood.

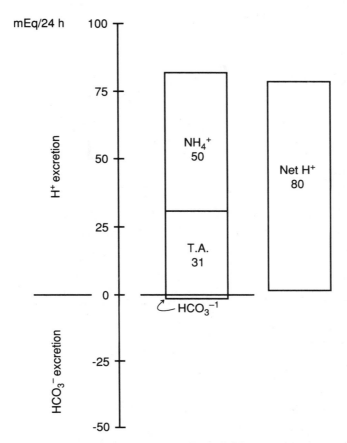

Fig. 6-2. Acid-base balance results in a constant total body HCO_3^- pool. In a person who produces 80 mEq of nonvolatile acid and loses 1 mEq of HCO_3^- in the urine per day acid-base balance is maintained by excreting in the urine 81 mEq of H^+ in the form of titratable acid (TA) and NH_4^+. The amount of HCO_3^- added to the HCO_3^- pool, or "net H^+ excretion," is given by the urinary TA and NH_4^+ minus the HCO_3^- lost in the urine, and it equals the daily production on nonvolatile acid.

Table 6-1 lists the most common causes of metabolic alkalosis and briefly describes the mechanism of alkalosis generation in different types of metabolic alkalosis.

MAINTENANCE OF A METABOLIC ALKALOSIS

Metabolic alkalosis will only persist if the body's HCO_3^- excess fails to be excreted and if the production rate and external loss of nonvolatile H^+ remain equal to each other.

The kidneys have a very large capacity to excrete HCO_3^-. Thus, the administration of 500 mEq of HCO_3^- daily to a normal person produces only the mildest form of metabolic alkalosis. However, metabolic alkalosis develops and persists in different disease states in spite of daily HCO_3^- addition rates of only 200 or 300 mEq. The reason for this is either that the ability of the kidneys to excrete the excess HCO_3^- is impaired, or that ongoing external H^+ losses equal the HCO_3^- losses.

Renal HCO_3^- reabsorption is a complex phenomenon involving several cellular ion transporting

Table 6-1.   Causes and Mechanisms of Generation of Metabolic Alkalosis

Clinical Syndrome	Mechanism Responsible for Generation of the Alkalosis	Urinary [Cl^-]
Vomiting, nasogastric suction	Negative H^+ balance due to external loss of gastric HCl	<15 mEq/L
Diuretic therapy	Negative H^+ balance due to increased urinary loss of H^+. Decreased space of distribution of HCO_3^-	<15 mEq/L (After diuretic wears off)
Congenital Cl^--wasting diarrhea, villous adenoma, laxatives	Negative H^+ balance due to increased rectal loss of H^+ as NH_4Cl. Decreased space of distribution of HCO_3^-	<15 mEq/L
Post-hypercapnia, nonreabsorbable anions (e.g., penicillin)	Body HCO_3^- excess or increased urinary H^+ loss combined to unavailability of exogenous Cl^-	<15 mEq/L
Primary (Low Renin) mineralocorticoid excess syndromes: primary hyperaldosteronism, DOC excess syndromes, Cushing's syndrome, mineralocorticoid-like agents (licorice)	Negative H^+ balance due to increased urinary loss of H^+, as NH_4Cl mainly. Magnitude of the alkalosis varies reciprocally with magnitude of coexisting K^+ deficit	>15 mEq/L
Secondary (low renin) mineralocorticoid excess syndromes: malignant HTN, renovascular HTN, reninomas	Same as above	>15 mEq/L
Bartters' syndrome, severe K^+ deficit (>800 mEq)	Defective tubular Cl^- reabsorption (resulting in increased urinary H^+ loss?)	>15 mEq/L
Alkali administration	Underlying renal failure predisposes to alkalosis	>15 mEq/L

steps. It normally amounts to some 4,500 mEq/day and it is also mediated through apical H^+ secretion. The proximal tubule reabsorbs 80% of the filtered HCO_3^-, the remaining 20% being reabsorbed by the loop of Henle, the distal tubule, and the collecting duct. The cellular mechanisms involved in HCO_3^- reabsorption are graphically depicted in Figure 6-3; the legend to that figure summarizes the manner of operation of those mechanisms.

The renal capacity to excrete a HCO_3^- load is impaired in most forms of metabolic alkalosis. This is due to the coexistence of other physiological perturbations that limit the ability of the kidney to excrete the excess HCO_3^-.

1. Extracellular fluid (ECF) volume depletion, which may act by (1) exclusively decreasing glomerular filtration rate (GFR), so that the filtered load of HCO_3^- remains normal or close to normal in the face of an increased serum [HCO_3^-]; (2) exclusively increasing the absolute amount of HCO_3^- reabsorbed by the tubules; and (3) a combination of decreased GFR and increased tubular HCO_3^- reabsorption.

A   B

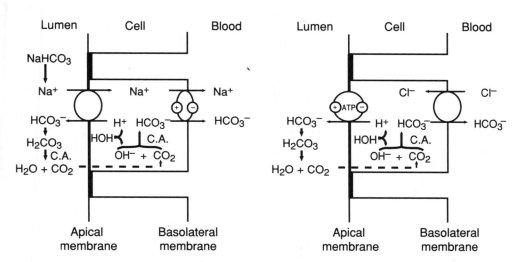

Fig. 6-3. (A & B) Graphic representation of the cellular mechanisms of urinary acidification as applied to the process of HCO_3^- reabsorption. The latter is actually mediated through secretion of H^+ into the lumen. The secreted H^+ reacts with luminal HCO_3^- to form H_2CO_3, which is then converted into CO_2 and H_2O; in the proximal tubule this conversion is accelerated by brush border carbonic anhydrase (CA). Notice that H^+ secretion does not actually result in luminal HCO_3^- reabsorption, but in addition of an equimolar amount of HCO_3^- to peritubular blood, as described in Figure 6-1.

(A) In proximal tubule cells apical H^+ secretion is mostly mediated by an electroneutral Na^+/H^+ antiporter that exchanges cell H^+ for luminal Na^+. Basolateral extrusion of HCO_3^- from the cell mainly occurs by electrogenic cotransport of HCO_3^- and Na^+, which results in depolarization of the basolateral cell membrane.

(B) Collecting duct luminal H^+ secretion exclusively occurs via an electrogenic proton ATPase located in the apical membrane of intercalated cells. Intercalated cell HCO_3^- extrusion takes place through a basolateral electroneutral Cl^-/HCO_3^- exchanger. A small fraction of proximal HCO_3^- reabsorption also proceeds through these cellular pathways. At least some intercalated cells in the collecting duct have the H^+ ATPase and Cl^-/HCO_3^- exchanger translocated to the basolateral and apical cell membranes, respectively. Consequently these cells are capable of secreting HCO_3^- into the urine in exchange for luminal Cl^-, a process which may be stimulated by systemic alkalosis.

2. Depletion of Cl^-, which could interfere with urinary loss of HCO_3^- through impaired anionic exchange of luminal Cl^- for cellular-peritubular HCO_3^-. The role of Cl^- depletion per se, independently of ECF volume depletion, in the maintenance of metabolic alkalosis is an extremely controversial matter.
3. Hypokalemia and K^+ depletion, which also enhance proximal and distal tubular HCO_3^- reabsorption. Hypokalemia is more important in maintaining the alkalosis of non–volume depleted states, such as the mineralocorticoid excess syndromes, than in the alkalosis due to vomiting and diuretics. Aldosterone and other adrenal steroids by themselves increase collecting duct H^+ secretion.
4. Elevated PCO_2 from "compensatory" hypoventilation, which increases renal H^+ secretion at either a low or a high blood pH.

Bicarbonaturia is the fastest pathway to the correction of metabolic alkalosis. However, metabolic alkalosis would also correct, albeit much slower, if the rate of external H^+ loss remained below the rate of nonvolatile H^+ production during a certain period of time. Thus, metabolic alkalosis persists in some circumstances because urinary H^+ output (particularly in the form of NH_4^+) fails to decrease. This might, for example, be due to sustained stimulation of H^+ secretion by diuretic agents or aldosterone.

DIAGNOSTIC APPROACH

When the cause of metabolic alkalosis is not clinically obvious, measurement of urinary Cl^- is often helpful in pointing toward the likely etiology. A low urinary Cl^- concentration (<15 mEq/L) is characteristic of conditions in which metabolic alkalosis coexists with ECF volume depletion, such as gastric HCl loss and diuretic use, and/or in which exogenous Cl^- is unavailable. On the other hand, a urinary Cl of greater than 51 mEq/L is typical, although not pathognomonic, of the mineralocorticoid excess syndromes. The behavior of urinary Cl in different types of metabolic alkalosis is also included in Table 6-1.

THERAPEUTIC APPROACH

In addition to its diagnostic role, urinary Cl is useful in guiding the management of patients with metabolic alkalosis. Thus, patients with low urinary Cl usually have "chloride-responsive" alkalosis, i.e., their alkalosis largely corrects when they are treated with solutions containing Cl^- in the form of NaCl. These solutions are thought to induce bicarbonaturia by replacing ECF volume deficits and/or Cl^- deficits.

When urinary Cl exceeds 15 mEq/L the metabolic alkalosis does not respond to treatment with NaCl. "Chloride resistance" occurs in metabolic alkalosis of any etiology when total body K^+ deficits reach 800 or more mEq, and in mineralocorticoid excess states. It responds to K^+ replacement, which may at times require the concomitant administration of KCl and a K^+-sparing diuretic, at least until the K^+ deficit is repaired. This maneuver results in bicarbonaturia and/or in a marked decrease in urinary net H^+ excretion, with correction of the alkalosis.

GENERAL READINGS

Cogan MG, Carneiro AV, Tatsuno J et al: Letter to the editor. J Am Soc Nephrol 1:1260, 1991

Good DW: New concepts in renal ammonium excretion. In Seldin DW, Giebisch G (eds): The Regulation of Acid-Base Balance. Raven Press, New York, 1989

Jakobson HR, Seldin DW: On the generation, maintenance, and correction of metabolic alkalosis. Am J Physiol 245:F425, 1983

Koeppen BM, Giebisch G: Segmental hydrogen ion transport. In Seldin DW, Giebisch G (eds): The Regulation of Acid-Base Balance. Raven Press, New York, 1989

Luke RG, Galla JH: Chloride-depletion alkalosis with a normal extracellular fluid volume. Am J Physiol 245: F419, 1983

Luke RG, Galla JH, Gifford JD: Effect of dietary chloride intake and the ability of the kidney to excrete a base load. J Am Soc Nephrol 1:1259, 1991

Sabatini S, Kurtzman NA: The maintenance of metabolic alkalosis: factors which decrease bicarbonate excretion. Kidney Int 25:357, 1984

Sabatini S, Kurtzman NA: Overall acid-base regulation by the kidney. In Seldin DW, Giebisch G (eds): The Regulation of Acid-Base Balance. Raven Press, New York, 1989

Seldin DW, Rector FC Jr: The generation and maintenance of metabolic alkalosis. Kidney Int 1:306, 1972

CASE STUDY 1

Alkalosis Associated with Vomiting

A 55-year-old man, Mr. Smith, experienced repeated vomiting and anorexia for four days. One week previously he had medicated himself with ibuprofen because of lower back aching. Although the vomiting had subsided he sought medical attention because of continuing anorexia and lightheadedness upon arising. The past medical history was insignificant.

PHYSICAL EXAMINATION

	Supine	Standing
B.P.	100/70 mmHg	90/60 mmHg
Pulse Rate	90	108
Respiratory Rate	10	
Temperature	98.8°F	
Weight	68 kg (baseline weight unknown)	

The physical examination was otherwise remarkable for mild epigastric tenderness and 1+ guaiac positive stools.

LABORATORY DATA

CBC

WBC 8,500/mm^3

HgB 16 gm/dL

PLT 292,000/mm^3

Serum Chemistry Panel

Na$^+$ 143 mEq/L	BUN 35 mg/dL
K$^+$ 3.0 mEq/L	Creatinine 1.7 mg/dL
Cl$^-$ 85 mEq/L	Total Prot. 8.5 gm/dL
Total CO$_2$ 39 mMols/L	Albumin 5.5 gm/dL

Urinalysis

Specific gravity: 1.018

Protein—Trace

Sediment—No formed elements

pH: 6.0

Question 1. Based on the history, physical findings, and initial laboratory results, how would you characterize the intravascular volume of this patient? What are your thoughts about the acid-base balance status of the patient?

Question 2. How would you explain the elevated anion gap of 19 mEq/L?

Question 3. How does vomiting actually result in metabolic alkalosis?

Question 4. If vomiting, which results in the net addition of 200 to 300 mEq of HCO$_3$$^-$ to body fluids a day, induces metabolic alkalosis, why does ingesting 500 mEq/day of NaHCO$_3$ fail to produce a significant metabolic alkalosis?

Question 5.   Why is the renal excretion of bicarbonate impaired after vomiting?

Question 6.   How does a decrease in ECF volume impair the ability of the kidneys to excrete bicarbonate?

Question 7.   How does a total body chloride deficit impair renal bicarbonate excretion?

Question 8.   What role does hypokalemia play in maintaining alkalosis?

Question 9.   Why is the hypoventilation that accompanies metabolic alkalosis a physiologic epiphenomenon of the alkalosis and not a truly compensatory mechanism?

---

1. **Based on the history, physical findings and initial laboratory results, how would you characterize the intravascular volume of this patient? What are your thoughts about the acid-base balance status of the patient?**

Volume depletion is suggested by the history of decreased oral intake, vomiting, lightheadedness and physical examination findings of borderline orthostatic changes in pulse rate and blood pressure. Laboratory data reveal decreased renal function, with an elevated BUN/creatinine ratio, also compatible with volume depletion. The history of vomiting, the elevated total CO_2, and the hypokalemia suggest that the patient has metabolic alkalosis. Actual confirmation of this diagnostic suspicion requires an arterial blood gas determination because sustained respiratory acidosis can also be associated with an elevated serum total CO_2.

An arterial blood gas is obtained and reveals the following values:

pH	7.52
PCO_2	46 mmHg
$[HCO_3^-]$	36 mEq/L

The arterial blood gas confirms that the patient has metabolic alkalosis. The PCO_2 is elevated because the alkalemia resulting from the high bicarbonate concentration decreases ventilation. As a result, in metabolic alkalosis the $PaCO_2$ increases by 0.7 to 0.9 mmHg (average increase of 0.8) for each 1 mEq/L increment in the plasma bicarbonate concentration.[1]

2. **How would you explain the elevated anion gap of 19 mEq/L?**

An increased anion gap is commonly seen in metabolic alkalosis, especially when the latter coexists with hypovolemia and hemoconcentration (e.g., vomiting or diuretics). Animal studies suggest that the anion gap increases in metabolic alkalosis by 5 mEq/L for each 0.1 pH unit increase.[2]

The increased anion gap in metabolic alkalosis results from two separate processes:

1. A modestly increased production of lactate (and possibly of other organic acids), due to the stimulation of phosphofructokinase by the alkalemia itself.[2]
2. An augmentation in the negative charges normally contributed by plasma proteins. This results from an increase in plasma protein concentration secondary to hemoconcentration, and an

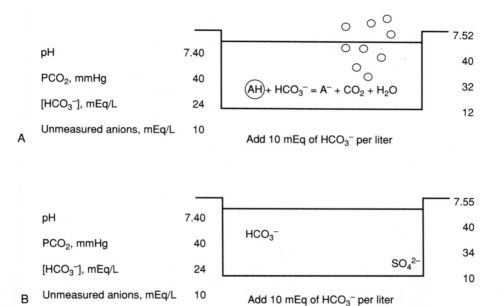

Fig. 6-4. (A) Addition of a fixed amount of HCO_3^- to a solution containing other buffers, as compared to (B) its addition to an unbuffered solution. A certain fraction of the added HCO_3^- reacts with protonated buffer, *AH*, and is thus dissipated into CO_2 gas, with a resulting increase in the concentration of dissociated buffer anion, A^-. The latter is, by definition, an "unmeasured anion."

increase in the net negative charge of individual protein molecules. The latter is related to the buffering effects of plasma proteins, as graphically explained in Figure 6-4.[2,3]

3. How does vomiting actually result in metabolic alkalosis?

When HCl is secreted into the lumen of the stomach, an equimolar amount of HCO_3^- is added to the blood (Fig. 6-5). As a consequence of this, the plasma Cl^- concentration decreases and the plasma HCO_3^- concentration increases.[4] This results in a minimal metabolic alkalosis of short duration, which is responsible for a transient alkalinization of the urine known as the "postprandial alkaline tide." The brief nature of this metabolic alkalosis is due to the emptying of the gastric acid contents into the duodenum. As HCl enters the duodenum, an equimolar amount of HCO_3^-, secreted into that bowel segment mainly by the pancreas, is titrated to CO_2 and H_2O[4]:

$$HCl + HCO_3^- \Leftrightarrow CO_2 + H_2O + Cl^- \qquad \text{(Eq. 6-3)}$$

Thus, the HCO_3^- previously added to the blood by the stomach is replaced mEq by mEq for Cl^- when HCO_3^--rich fluids are secreted into the duodenum. The entire process results in a recycling of the two main plasma anions across the gastrointestinal wall without a sustained change in the anionic composition of the plasma.

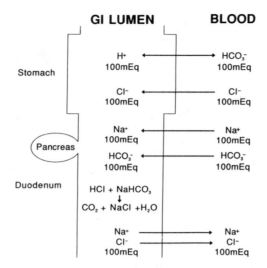

Fig. 6-5. The secretion of 100 mEq of H^+ as HCl by the stomach results in the replacement of 100 mEq of plasma Cl^- for 100 mEq of HCO_3^-. The pancreas restores the anionic composition of plasma to normal by secreting 100 mEq of HCO_3^- into the duodenum in the form of $NaHCO_3$. Neutralization of gastric HCl by pancreatic $NaHCO_3$ in the duodenum transforms the luminal contents into NaCl, a neutral salt absorbed without any effect on systemic acid-base balance. External loss of gastric HCl through vomiting disrupts the above cycle and results in net addition of HCO_3^- to the blood.

The external loss of gastric HCl through vomiting or a physiologically equivalent mechanism (nasogastric suction, gastrostomy drainage) disrupts the anion recycling process described above. The HCO_3^- added to the blood during gastric HCl secretion is no longer titrated by HCl entering the small bowel. As a result, there is an enrichment of body fluids with HCO_3^-, together with an equimolar depletion of Cl^-. Vomiting may thus result in the net addition of 200 to 300 mEq of HCO_3^- to body fluids a day.

4. **If vomiting, which results in the net addition of 200 to 300 mEq of HCO_3^- to body fluids a day, induces metabolic alkalosis, why does ingesting 500 mEq/day of $NaHCO_3$ fail to produce a significant metabolic alkalosis?**

Ingesting 500 mEq of bicarbonate does not significantly raise the plasma $[HCO_3^-]$ because the kidneys excrete the ingested bicarbonate.[5] By contrast, the kidney fails to excrete the bicarbonate generated by vomiting and, henceforth, metabolic alkalosis develops.

5. **Why is the renal excretion of bicarbonate impaired after vomiting?**

Vomiting is associated with several physiologic perturbations. These perturbations, which do not occur during bicarbonate administration, impair the ability of the kidneys to excrete a bicarbonate load. They include: (1) ECF volume depletion, (2) a deficit in total body chloride, (3) hypokalemia, and (4) a compensatory elevation of the PCO_2.

To understand why metabolic alkalosis persists we must understand how the physiologic perturbations accompanying vomiting interfere with renal bicarbonate excretion.

6. How does a decrease in ECF volume impair the ability of the kidneys to excrete bicarbonate?

ECF volume depletion (ECFVD) enhances proximal tubular Na and bicarbonate reabsorption. Additionally, ECFVD often results in a decrease in GFR. Further, ECFVD increases aldosterone secretion, which augments distal nephron H^+ secretion and bicarbonate reabsorption.

The relative roles of a decreased GFR and of an increase in tubular bicarbonate reabsorption in maintaining the metabolic alkalosis associated with ECFVD will be discussed first. It will then be explained how the physiologic controls of several cellular mechanisms responsible for HCO_3^- reabsorption may be modified by both the metabolic alkalosis itself and the associated ECFVD so as to result in an increased renal HCO_3^- reabsorptive capacity.

Volume Depletion and a Decreased GFR

The filtered load of bicarbonate is equal to the product of the GFR $\times$ Plasma $[HCO_3^-]$. When vomiting occurs, the elevated plasma bicarbonate concentration tends to increase the filtered load of bicarbonate, while the decrease in GFR has the opposite effect. As a result, the filtered load of bicarbonate in metabolic alkalosis varies depending on what happens to GFR. Consequently, the process of maintenance of the alkalosis does not *necessarily* imply that the kidneys are reabsorbing a larger than normal amount of bicarbonate.

In some animal models of metabolic alkalosis, GFR may be spared, while in other models it is decreased.[6–8] Consequently the maintenance of metabolic alkalosis may be associated with either an increased, normal, or even a decreased rate of HCO_3^- reabsorption by the tubules, depending on the behavior of GFR. Human research data indicate that the elevated serum HCO_3^- concentration achieved by gastric aspiration is not accompanied by a proportional reduction in GFR. This results in an increased filtered load of HCO_3^-.[9] Therefore, in order for metabolic alkalosis to be maintained in humans following gastric aspiration, the absolute amount of bicarbonate reabsorbed by the tubules must be increased. However, complementary experiments suggest that there may be an upper limit to the amount of HCO_3^- that can be reabsorbed by the human kidney.[10] The data suggest that hypercarbonatemia in excess of 33 mEq/L can only persist if GFR is decreased.[10]

It is accepted that absolute bicarbonate reabsorption, i.e., the number of mEq of HCO_3^- reabsorbed by the kidneys per unit of time, is markedly increased in some experimental models of alkalosis. This indicates that at least some of the cellular mechanisms responsible for bicarbonate reabsorption normally operate well below their maximal rate capacities.[11]

In clinical metabolic alkalosis due to vomiting, the filtered bicarbonate load may be increased if GFR is relatively spared. In this situation the metabolic alkalosis is sustained through an increase in absolute tubular bicarbonate reabsorption, i.e., in the number of mEq of HCO_3^- reabsorbed per unit of time. Patients with the most severe form of vomiting-induced metabolic alkalosis have pronounced azotemia, i.e., markedly reduced GFR. Under these conditions the filtered load of bicarbonate can be normal or decreased. These patients maintain their metabolic alkalosis by reabsorbing an absolute amount of bicarbonate equal to or less than that reabsorbed by the kidneys of normal individuals.

Volume Depletion and Increased Tubular Bicarbonate Reabsorption

The elevated serum $[HCO_3^-]$ per se influences proximal HCO_3^- reabsorption in opposite directions during metabolic alkalosis. On the one hand, luminal HCO_3^- concentration increases and results in augmented proximal tubular HCO_3^- reabsorption. This is due to the increased buffering power of the tubular fluid, which favors H^+ secretion by maintaining a relatively high luminal pH. On the other hand, the elevated pH and $[HCO_3^-]$ of peritubular blood and tubular cells inhibit proximal HCO_3^- reabsorption.[11–13]

Superimposed upon the effects of the elevated $[HCO_3^-]$ itself are the physiologic perturbations accompanying vomiting, especially ECF volume depletion, which shift the balance in favor of increased HCO_3^- reabsorption. Vomiting-induced volume depletion increases proximal HCO_3^- reabsorption through two different mechanisms. First, volume depletion increases the levels of angiotensin II, which is a powerful stimulus of the Na^+/H^+ exchanger.[14] This stimulation results in an increased rate of luminal HCO_3^- removal (Fig. 6-6). Second, volume depletion decreases the normally existing blood-to-lumen backleak of HCO_3^-.[11] This maximizes net HCO_3^- reabsorption for any given rate of luminal bicarbonate removal (Fig. 6-6).

Apart from its effects on the proximal tubule, volume depletion results in an increase in aldosterone secretion. Aldosterone stimulates H^+ secretion and bicarbonate reabsorption by the cortical collecting duct.[14]

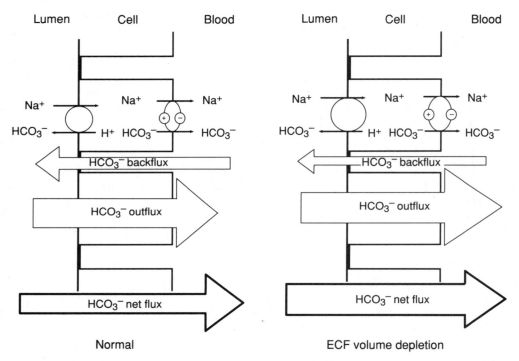

Fig. 6-6. Effects of volume depletion on proximal HCO_3^- reabsorption. Normally some of the HCO_3^- extruded through the basolateral cell membrane (HCO_3^- outflux) diffuses back into the lumen via the lateral intercellular spaces and tight junctions (HCO_3^- backflux). The actual amount of HCO_3^- being reabsorbed, of HCO_3^- net flux, is the difference between HCO_3^- outflux and backflux.

ECF volume depletion results in stimulation of the renin-angiotensin system. Angiotensin II, a powerful stimulus of the apical Na^+/H^+ antiporter, is responsible for increased HCO_3^- outflux in volume-depleted states; this is graphically depicted by the larger size of the antiporter. At the same time volume depletion decreases paracellular (intercellular) backflux of Na^+ salts, thus contributing to increase net HCO_3^- reabsorption.

7. How does a total body chloride deficit impair renal bicarbonate excretion?

During gastric HCl losses chloride depletion is soon followed by volume depletion. Early on, when HCl loss first occurs, bicarbonaturia ensues and there is a concomitant naturiesis and kaliuresis, as well as a marked increase in urine pH to values of 7 and above.[15] This kaliuresis (and not the rather small gastric K^+ losses) is responsible for the status of negative K^+ balance and hypokalemia that typically accompany the alkalosis. Chloride, however, disappears from the urine immediately, and the urinary $[Cl^-]$ is less than 15 mEq/L.[15] Thus, in this situation urinary $[Cl^-]$ may be a more sensitive indicator of ECFVD than urinary $[Na^+]$.[16]

With persistent vomiting and decreased oral intake, the bicarbonaturia and natiuresis cease and the kaliuresis decreases, although urinary K^+ still remains inappropriately high.[15] It is at this point that the urine pH becomes acidic again (pH of 6 or less). This is the classic "paradoxical aciduria" seen in the presence of systemic alkalemia and metabolic alkalosis.

From the standpoint of urinary electrolyte composition, metabolic alkalosis due to vomiting is characterized by the disappearance of practically all chloride from the urine. This occurs throughout both the development (early) and the maintenance (late) phases of the alkalosis.

The virtual disappearance of Cl^- from the urine is of crucial diagnostic help in ascertaining the etiology of metabolic alkalosis in "subreptitious vomiters." These patients present with hypokalemia and metabolic alkalosis. Some of them maintain an oral intake high enough to prevent the occurrence of major volume depletion, so that their urine remains alkaline and sustained natriuresis and kaliuresis exist. Despite the bicarbonaturia, they still maintain the alkalosis because their combined nonvolatile H^+ production plus urinary HCO_3^- excretion is largely equal to their daily gastric HCl losses.

In most cases, however, metabolic alkalosis persists because bicarbonaturia first decreases and then abates. Why does the bicarbonaturia abate? One reason is that ECF volume depletion limits bicarbonate excretion through the mechanisms already described above. A separate reason could be that chloride depletion, reflected in the very low urinary $[Cl^-]$, could by itself interfere with urinary bicarbonate excretion by limiting chloride availability in specific nephron segments. A major unresolved controversy exists regarding whether chloride depletion impairs the capacity of the kidneys to excrete bicarbonate independently of ECF volume depletion.[17,18]

Urinary electrolytes were measured in the patient under discussion and revealed:

$$
\begin{array}{ll}
U\,[Na^+] & 7 \text{ mEq/L} \\
U\,[K^+] & 25 \text{ mEq/L} \\
U\,[Cl^-] & 3 \text{ mEq/L} \\
U\,pH & 6
\end{array}
$$

These results confirm the presence of paradoxical aciduria and marked avidity not only for Cl^- but also for Na^+, thus indicating a significant degree of ECFVD.

Effects of Chloride Depletion on Renal Bicarbonate Handling

In normal individuals a decreased Cl^- intake impairs excretion of HCO_3^- and thus predisposes to a persistant metabolic alkalosis whenever negative H^+ balance occurs.[19] This phenomenon most likely accounts for the metabolic alkalosis that develops when Cl^- intake is limited after the correction of hypercapnia, or during the administration of large amounts of nonreabsorbable anions, such as certain penicillins. The main questions surrounding the effects of Cl^- is where in the nephron Cl^- deficiency interferes with HCO_3^- excretion, and if it is possible to physiologically separate a Cl^- from an ECF volume deficit.

It is now clear that a subpopulation of intercalated cells in the cortical collecting duct is capable of secreting HCO_3^- into the lumen in exchange for Cl^-.[11,14] Some experimental data suggest that in metabolic alkalosis, reduced delivery of chloride to the collecting duct impairs urinary excretion of bicarbonate by interfering with collecting duct bicarbonate secretion.[20-24] However, other investigators have concluded that simply increasing chloride delivery to the collecting duct does not achieve a bicarbonaturia in metabolic alkalosis.[25-27] According to this group of investigators significant bicarbonaturia only occurs when the delivery of bicarbonate to the distal nephron is increased.[26] Such an increase in distal HCO_3^- delivery can be accomplished during ECF volume expansion with Cl^--containing solutions through an increase in GFR, an inhibition of proximal HCO_3^- reabsorption, or a combination of both. The main reason for the bicarbonaturia would then be increased distal bicarbonate delivery, and not just collecting duct bicarbonate secretion.[27]

This controversy does not exclude the possibility that slow correction of metabolic alkalosis might occur through a decrease in collecting duct *net* H^+ secretion.[21] The latter may be thought of as representing the net balance between the H^+ and HCO_3^- being simultaneously secreted by the collecting duct (and also possibly by different segments of that duct). Obviously that balance could be crucially dependent upon delivery of Cl^- to the cortical collecting duct, where it mediates HCO_3^- secretion.

From a practical standpoint, chloride and volume depletion coexist in vomiting-induced metabolic alkalosis. Using a black box approach it is evident that restoration of body fluid volume and total electrolyte content and composition to normal requires replacing both chloride and volume deficits. This is true independent of any role chloride may play in correcting the alkalosis via a specific intrarenal mechanism, e.g. collecting duct chloride–bicarbonate exchange.

8. What role does hypokalemia play in maintaining metabolic alkalosis?

Renal tubular hydrogen ion secretion and bicarbonate reabsorption are enhanced by hypokalemia. This phenomenon occurs in both proximal tubule and distal nephron segments, although the exact mechanisms involved may be different at these two sites.[28-30]

To what degree hypokalemia contributes to the maintenance of clinical metabolic alkalosis associated with volume depletion remains unclear. In patients with metabolic alkalosis induced by HCl depletion, the administration of NaCl, without repair of K deficits, largely corrects the alkalosis.[20,31] However, K depletion seems to play a crucial role in maintaining the metabolic alkalosis associated with mineralocorticoid excess states, which cannot be corrected without repair of the K deficits.[20] These findings are consistent with the view that hypokalemia plays less of a role in maintaining metabolic alkalosis in volume depleted (e.g., vomiting) as compared to volume expanded states (e.g., mineralocorticoid excess).

9. Why is the hypoventilation that accompanies metabolic alkalosis a physiologic epiphenomenon of the alkalosis and not a truly "compensatory" mechanism?

In respiratory acidosis, the increased arterial PCO_2 stimulates H^+ secretion and results in the net addition of bicarbonate to body fluids. Moreover, the elevated PCO_2 enhances renal bicarbonate reabsorption and thus prevents the urinary excretion of the newly generated bicarbonate.

As mentioned earlier, metabolic alkalosis induces "compensatory" hypoventilation and thus results in an elevated PCO_2. In experimental animals this elevation in the PCO_2 has similar effects on renal H^+ secretion in both metabolic alkalosis and respiratory acidosis; i.e., the generation of new bicarbonate, which is added to body fluids. For this reason, the plasma HCO_3^- concentration is higher when PCO_2 is allowed to "compensatorily" rise than when it is not.[32]

Interestingly, in the above experiments the elevated blood pH was minimally reduced by the "compensatory" PCO_2 elevation. This is because the elevation in plasma $[HCO_3^-]$ resulting from the renal effects of the compensatory hypercapnia is nearly exactly proportional to the degree of PCO_2 elevation (Fig. 6-7). This phenomenon illustrates how the hypoventilation of metabolic alkalosis is not a physiologic mechanism geared to normalize blood pH. That is, it is not a truly compensatory phenomenon, but rather the inevitable physiologic response to an alkaline pH shift in the region of the respiratory center.[1]

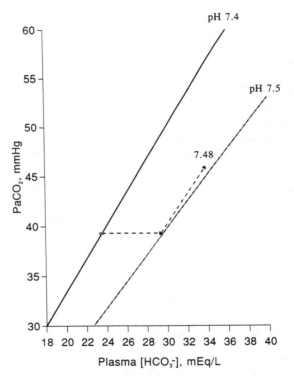

Fig. 6-7. As a consequence of an elevation in plasma $[HCO_3^-]$ from 24 to 30 mEq/L the $PaCO_2$ rises from 40 to 46 mmHg. This increase in $PaCO_2$ stimulates renal H^+ secretion and results in addition of new HCO_3^- to body fluids. The plasma $[HCO_3^-]$ increases further, to 34 mEq/L, and for this reason blood pH stays practically the same as if the $PaCO_2$ had not risen (7.48 vs. 7.50). (Modified from Nicolaos,[32] with permission.)

Therapeutic Implications

When confronted with a given patient there are usually uncertainties surrounding the relative importance of the above discussed factors in maintaining the alkalosis. A very common therapeutic plan involves simultaneously correcting all possible abnormalities, including volume, chloride, and K deficits.

The measurement of urinary Cl^- is very helpful in assessing the potential for a therapeutic response to volume expansion with NaCl-containing solutions. This treatment is likely to largely correct the alkalosis when urinary $[Cl^-]$ is less than 15 mEq/L (chloride-responsive metabolic alkalosis), but not when it is higher.

Chloride-resistant metabolic alkalosis is characterized by a urinary $[Cl^-]$ greater than 15 mEq/L and is typical (although not pathognomonic) of the primary mineralocorticoid excess syndromes. In these cases, sustained correction of the alkalosis can only be accomplished by replacing the K^+ deficit. It so happens that very profound total K^+ deficits of any etiology (800 mEq or more) may by themselves prevent the kidneys from restoring body composition to normal in patients with hypovolemic metabolic alkalosis.[33] The severe K^+ depletion impairs the ability of the kidney to maximally reabsorb Cl^-.[34,35] In this situation the administration of NaCl solutions fails to achieve the expected restoration of ECF volume. Consequently, the large bicarbonaturia required to correct the alkalosis does not occur until the K^+ deficit is at least partially corrected. This supports the clinician's wisdom that in hypovolemic metabolic alkalosis replacing all existing deficits effects correction of the alkalosis.

Patients who have effective instead of factual ECF volume depletion are usually edematous (heart failure, decompensated cirrhosis) and should not be treated with NaCl-containing solutions. They can be given Cl^- in the form of KCl, but there is a limit to how much KCl they can tolerate without becoming hyperkalemic before the alkalosis is corrected. In these patients, combining KCl and the carbonic anhydrase inhibitor acetazolamide often achieves a large bicarbonaturia and correction of the alkalosis. If this fails, the alkalosis may be corrected by infusion of 150 millimolar HCl (or an HCl precursor, such as NH_4Cl, lysine, or arginine hydrochloride) into a *major* vein. In patients with renal failure, metabolic alkalosis can also be corrected by dialysis against a bath containing 20 to 25 mEq/L of bicarbonate.

Finally it must be understood that efforts should be made whenever possible to prevent the development of metabolic alkalosis. Thus, it should be remembered metabolic alkalosis is seen much less often now than just 20 years ago, especially in surgical wards. This is largely due to the administration of H_2 antagonists to patients undergoing gastric aspiration, with the result that gastric drainage is no longer synonymous with large losses of HCl.

CASE STUDY 2

Alkalosis Associated with Hypertension

Dr. Uhuru, a pleasant 38-year-old female space engineer, presented to her physician because of "leg tiredness after climbing ten steps." Her past medical history was remarkable for two uncomplicated pregnancies (G2P2, last delivery at age 34) with a questionable history of mild HTN 2 years before this visit. Review of systems was remarkable for nocturia over the last 3 months, despite her avoidance of fluids in the evenings. She did not ingest prescribed or OTC medications, did not smoke, and drank alcohol occasionally. She described her diet as a "normal" American diet.

PHYSICAL EXAMINATION

	Supine	Standing
B.P.	178/112 mmHg	156/94 mmHg
Heart Rate	86	92

Weight 57 kg
Possibe trace of ankle edema
Rapid fatigability of the limbs muscles, confirmed after
repetitive motion against an applied resistance

LABORATORY DATA
Spun hematocrit 36
Urinalysis (Fasting A.M. UA): 0 WBC/RBC; pH 7.0–7.5 by dipstick; trace proteinuria
Specific gravity 1.012

Question 1.   Based on the history, physical findings, and the provided laboratory
data, what do you think may be wrong with the patient? Which other
laboratory tests would you order and why?

Question 2.   How would you interpret the above results, and what further questions
would you ask the patient?

Question 3.   How would you proceed next?

Question 4.   The urine pH in this patient has to be very close to the blood pH, so
her urine must contain a certain amount of bicarbonate and cannot
contain much titratable acid (TA). How can she maintain the metabolic
alkalosis when in addition to not excreting any TA she loses bicarbonate in the urine?

Question 5.   When the patient was given salt tablets, her hypokalemia and metabolic alkalosis worsened. Would you have expected this if she has primary hyperaldosteronism?

Question 6.   Provide a more integrated view of how metabolic alkalosis develops
and is maintained in primary mineralocorticoid excess syndromes.

---

1. **Based on the history, physical findings and the provided laboratory data, what
do you think may be wrong with the patient? Which other laboratory tests would
you order and why?**

The pertinent findings are the following: recent onset of hypertension with an orthostatic fall in
blood pressure; nocturia with a nearly isosthenuria urine (urine SG after overnight fast that is
practically equal to the SG of plasma); and muscle fatigability and/or weakness. The triad of
hypertension, nocturia, and isosthenuria constitutes a classic form of presentation of chronic
renal failure. Nocturia is due to a concentrating defect and can be an early sign of renal insufficiency. Although the normal hematocrit makes it unlikely that severe renal insufficiency is present, the BUN and serum creatinine concentrations should be measured.

Confirmed muscle fatigue or weakness in a hypertensive patient should make one suspect the possibility of hypokalemia. The fasting alkaline urine could be a clue to the presence of a systemic alkalosis, which often coexists with hypokalemia. Additionally, hypokalemia can interfere with the renal concentrating mechanism and lead to nocturia. Therefore, the next step should be to measure the serum electrolytes. If hypokalemia is present measuring the urine electrolytes provides a clue about the origin of the hypokalemia.

Serum Electrolytes and Renal Chemistries

Na^+ 146 mEq/L	Cl^- 98 mEq/L
K^+ 2.8 mEq/L	BUN/Creatinine 10/0.9 mg/dL
HCO_3^- 36 mEq/L	

Urine Electrolytes

Na^+ 67 mEq/L
K^+ 27 mEq/L
Cl^- 80 mEq/L

---

2. How would you interpret these results and what further questions would you ask the patient?

The striking abnormalities are: (1) hypokalemia with an inappropriately high urinary K, suggesting that the hypokalemia is of renal origin; (2) mild hypernatremia; (3) elevated total CO_2 (which in the absence of a history of smoking or lung disease favors metabolic alkalosis rather than respiratory acidosis); (4) a high urinary chloride, which does not favor vomiting or other gastrointestinal origin of the alkalosis; and (5) the urinary $[Na^+]$ greater than 20 mEq/L argues against the patient being volume depleted.

The most common cause of hypokalemia and alkalosis in a hypertensive patient is diuretic use. It is possible (but not likely) that a hypertensive patient may become hypokalemic due to diarrhea, even surreptitious vomiting, or diuretic or laxative abuse. However, when asked the patient denied diuretic or laxative use, did not have any GI dysfunction and had a high urinary $[Cl^-]$. This certainly could be caused by diuretic drugs. Although she seemed to be a well-balanced person, if there is a question about surreptitious diuretic use the urine should be tested for diuretic drugs. Hypertension rules out, by definition, Bartter syndrome. Otherwise, the association of hypokalemia and hypertension makes a mineralocorticoid excess or a physiologically closely related syndrome most likely.[35–39] She laughed when asked if she had any passion for British licorice.

3. How would you proceed next?

It is possible that when first seen the patient was recovering from an acute viral illness, e.g., gastroenteritis. On the other hand, mineralocorticoid excess syndromes are chronic conditions. Confirmation of the previous laboratory abnormalities would be useful in establishing that the patient has an ongoing process and that she is in some form of steady state.

	Serum		Urine
Na$^+$ 144 mEq/L	HCO$_3^-$ 36 mEq/L		pH 7.5
K$^+$ 2.7 mEq/L	BUN 11 mg/dL		K$^+$ 30
Cl$^-$ 96 mEq/L	Creatinine 0.8 mg/dL		Na$^+$ 65
			Cl$^-$ 81
			SG 1.011

Arterial Blood Gas: pH: 7.48; PCO$_2$: 46 mmHg; [HCO$_3^-$]: 33 mEq/L

Since the previously observed electrolyte abnormalities persist, it is very likely that the patient has a mineralocorticoid excess syndrome. Confirmation of this can be done in different manners. In this case it was decided to have the patient fast after 6 P.M. and to administer 40 mg of p.o. furosemide at night and 40 mg the next morning, after which she will report to the office for plasma renin determinations.

4. The urine pH in this patient has to be very close to the blood pH, so her urine must contain a certain amount of bicarbonate and cannot contain much titratable acid (TA). How can she maintain the metabolic alkalosis when in addition to not excreting any TA she loses bicarbonate in the urine?

This question is a very pertinent and intriguing one. No one would argue that the urine of this patient contains very little, if any, TA. In addition, it is likely to contain 20 or more mEq/L of bicarbonate. On her usual diet she will make the customary amount of nonvolatile H$^+$, let us say, 65 mEq per day; in addition she will lose about 50 mEq of HCO$_3^-$ daily in her isosthenuric urine. In order to maintain her serum [HCO$_3^-$] constant she has to generate some 115 (65 + 50) mEq of HCO$_3^-$. Could her kidneys be doing this? The answer is *yes:* her 24-hour urine is practically certain to contain about 115 mmols of NH$_4^+$, which, given its pK$_a'$ of 9.2, may occur in high concentration in alkaline urines (Fig. 6-8). Such an amount of NH$_4^+$ is well within the ammoniogenic capacity of the kidney, which happens to be stimulated by hypokalemia.[40]

Results of Special Tests and Follow-up Comments
Upon completion of her post-furosemide plasma renin test, she was given NaCl tablets to take, at a total dose of 120 mmol daily for 1 week. She was told to maintain a high intake of citrus fruits and juices. The plasma renin results were as follows:

Pre-furosemide weight: 57 kg   post-furosemide weight: 55 kg
Both supine and erect post-furosemide plasma renin activities are below the lower limits of
     normal.
A random serum cortisol is within the low normal range.

These results indicate that the patient has a suppressed plasma renin, which cannot be stimulated by diuretic-induced volume depletion. This makes almost certain that she has a primary mineralocorticoid excess syndrome; hyperaldosteronism is the most likely one in her case. Thus, she is instructed to collect a 24-hour urine sample for Na and aldosterone determinations during

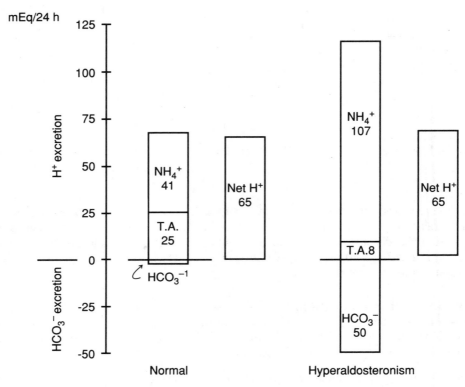

Fig. 6-8. Net acid excretion remains normal in primary hyperaldosteronism even though the urine is alkaline and contains relatively large amounts of HCO_3^-. Under these conditions, it is still possible to excrete large amounts of H^+ in the form of NH_4^+, which, given its pK_a' of 9.2, remains largely protonated in an alkaline urine.

her last day on NaCl tablets. The following morning her weight is 57.25 kg and her blood pressure is 186/114 mmHg in the sitting position. Her serum electrolytes are as follows:

Na^+ 147 mEq/L CO_2 41 mmol/L
K^+ 2.1 mEq/L   BUN 8 mg/dL
Cl^- 95 mEq/L   Creatinine 0.8 mg/dL

She is now asked to follow a low-salt (3 gm Na) diet and to continue her high ingestion of citrus fruits and juices. She is also started on KCl tablets, at a total dose of 64 mmols/day. She is requested to return to the office in 4 days for blood pressure and laboratory follow-up. When she returns her weight is 56.5 kg, her sitting blood pressure 154/98 mmHg and her serum chemistries are the following:

Na^+ 143 mEq/L CO_2 31 mmol/L
K^+ 3.6mEq/L   BUN 12 mg/dL
Cl^- 101 mEq/L   Creatinine 0.8 mg/dL

The 24-hour urine, collected while on NaCl supplements, contained 275 mEq of Na^+ and more than twice the upper limit of the amount of aldosterone excreted by normal persons consuming a regular diet. Clearly the high-salt diet failed to inhibit the secretion of aldosterone. The patient is told that she has a condition called primary hyperaldosteronism and referred to an endocrinologist for further work-up, given the possibility that her condition may be surgically curable.

5. When the patient was given salt tablets, her hypokalemia and metabolic alkalosis worsened. Would you have expected this if she has primary hyperaldosteronism?

High salt intake aggravates the hypokalemia of primary mineralocorticoid excess syndromes.[41] This is due to the fact that patients with primary hyperaldosteronismin are chronically volume expanded and very rapidly excrete a salt load. To do this their delivery of Na^+-rich fluid to the cortical collecting duct is increased. Given the high levels of aldosterone, this results in a major increase in the rate of K^+ secretion and renal K^+ loss.[42]

The ECF volume expansion of patients with primary hyperaldosteronism is most likely responsible for the observation that their urine is often alkaline and contains significant amounts of bicarbonate.[36,38,39] In the patient under discussion, the high-salt diet, which one could expect might increase bicarbonaturia and thus ameliorate the alkalosis, not only worsened the hypokalemia but also the metabolic alkalosis.

The above observation probably should be linked to another follow-up finding: that the metabolic alkalosis improved when serum K^+ rose in response to a low-Na diet and oral KCl supplementation. In patients with primary hyperaldosteronism there is a significant inverse correlation between the serum K^+ and serum HCO_3^- concentrations.[42] In the absence of significant hypokalemia, hypoaldosteronism only induces a very mild elevation in the serum $[HCO_3^-]$, 3 or 4 mEq/L at most. This may account for the observation that normal individuals given aldosterone in doses high enough to simulate hyperaldosteronism only develop very mild alkalosis.[42]

6. I understand how in hyperaldosteronism a significant degree of metabolic alkalosis can be maintained, even if the urine is alkaline, through an increased urinary excretion of NH_4^+. I also remember that aldosterone increases distal nephron H^+ secretion. On the other hand, I am now told that in hyperaldosteronism significant metabolic alkalosis only develops when hypokalemia is severe. **Provide a more integrated view of how metabolic alkalosis develops and is maintained in primary mineralocorticoid excess syndromes.**

Unfortunately it is not possible to explain with certainty how hyperaldosteronism results in sustained elevations in serum $[HCO_3^-]$ to values greater than 30 mEq/L, and how hypokalemia interacts with the elevated levels of aldosterone to achieve the alkalosis. The following explanation should only be taken as a plausible sequence of events.

In primary hyperaldosteronism renal net acid excretion is subject to two opposing influences. On one hand, the high aldosterone level enhances distal nephron H^+ secretion and HCO_3^- reabsorption. On the other hand, the high levels of aldosterone induce a status of chronic ECF volume expansion, which in turn results in an inhibition of more proximal HCO_3^- reabsorption, and increased delivery of HCO_3^- to the distal nephron. If the distal HCO_3^- delivery is so high that the distal HCO_3^- load cannot be fully reabsorbed by the aldosterone-stimulated collecting duct, bicarbonate will spill into the urine. The alkalosis will then improve. Hypokalemia increases proximal HCO_3^- reabsorption, thus opposing the effects of ECF volume expansion.[28,29]

It should be remembered that for metabolic alkalosis to *develop* net acid loss (i.e., HCO_3^- gain) *must* exceed net acid production. For metabolic alkalosis to be *maintained* net acid loss only needs to equal again net acid production. In addition, if GFR is spared, the net rate of H^+ secretion by the kidneys must also be elevated since plasma HCO_3^- is by definition elevated.

In hyperaldosteronism, bicarbonaturia has a moderating effect on the severity of the alkalosis. On the other hand, hypokalemia has an aggravating effect on the alkalosis and the severity of the alkalosis depends on the degree of hypokalemia.[43] Thus, hypokalemia must act by increasing net acid loss, making the difference between acid loss and acid production larger. This could be mediated through an increase in proximal and/or distal HCO_3^- reabsorption, as mentioned above.

Alternatively, the effect of hypokalemia may also relate to its role in enhancing proximal tubular NH_4^+ secretion. It must be remembered that in order to maintain a normal or elevated net acid excretion in an alkaline urine, as it happens in primary hyperaldosteronism, a large urinary excretion rate of NH_4^+ is required, and this may be crucially dependent upon the magnitude of the K^+ deficit. Taken altogether, it seems that the separation between the processes responsible for the generation and for the maintenance of the alkalosis in hyperaldosteronism is far less clear than that ideally compatible with best didactics. From the therapeutic standpoint, however, correction of K^+ deficits is a must for the correction of the alkalosis. Potassium-sparing diuretics are often required in these situations, often together with K^+ supplementation, especially during the initial phase of treatment.

REFERENCES

1. Javaheri S, Kazemi H: Metabolic alkalosis and hypoventilation in humans. Am Rev Respir Dis 136: 1011, 1987
2. Gabow PA: Disorders associated with an altered anion gap. Kidney Int 27:472, 1985
3. Madias NE, Ayus JC, Adrogue HJ: Increased anion gap in metabolic alkalosis. N Engl J Med 300: 1421, 1979
4. Charney AL, Feldman GM: Internal exchange of hydrogen ions: the gastrointestinal tract. In Seldin DW, Giebisch G (eds): Regulation of Acid-Base Balance. Raven Press, New York, 1989
5. Van Goidsenhoven M-T, Gray OV, Price AV, Sanderson PH: The effect of prolonged administration of large doses of sodium bicarbonate in man. Clin Sci 13:383, 1954
6. Borkan S, Northrup TE, Cohen JJ, Garella S: Renal response to metabolic alkalosis induced by isovolemic hemofiltration in the dog. Kidney Int 32:322, 1987
7. Cogan MG, Liu F-Y: Metabolic alkalosis in the rat. J Clin Invest 71:1141, 1983
8. Maddox DA, Gennari FJ: Proximal tubular bicarbonate reabsorption and PCO_2 in chronic metabolic alkalosis in the rat. J Clin Invest 72:1385, 1983
9. Berger BE, Cogan MG, Sebastian A: Reduced glomerular filtration and enhanced bicarbonate reabsorption maintain metabolic alkalosis in humans. Kidney Int 26:205, 1984
10. Vaz Carneiro A, Sebastian A, Cogan MG: Reduced glomerular filtration rate can maintain a rise in plasma bicarbonate concentration in humans. Am J Nephrol 7:450, 1987
11. Koeppen BM, Giebisch G: Segmental hydrogen ion transport. In Seldin DW, Giebisch G (eds): The Regulation of Acid-Base Balance. Raven Press, New York, 1989
12. Akiba T, Rocco VK, Warnock DG: Parallel adaptation of the rabbit renal cortical sodium/proton antiporter and sodium/bicarbonate cotransporter in metabolic acidosis and alkalosis. J Clin Invest 80:308, 1987
13. Liu F-Y, Cogan MG: Angiotensin II: a potent regulator of acidification in the rat early proximal convoluted tubule. J Clin Invest 80:272, 1987
14. Levine DZ, Jacobson HR: The regulation of renal acid secretion: new observations from studies of distal nephron segments. Kidney Int 29:1099, 1986
15. Kassirer JP, Schwartz WB: The response of normal man to selective depletion of hydrochloric acid. Am J Med 40:10, 1966
16. Kamel KS, Ethier JH, Richardson RMA et al: Urine electrolytes and osmolality: when and how to use them. Am J Nephrol 10:89, 1990

17. Luke RG, Galla JH, Gifford JD: To the editor: effect of dietary chloride intake and the ability of the kidney to excrete a base load. J Am Soc Nephrol 1:1259, 1991
18. Cogan MG, Carneiro AV, Tatsuno J et al: To the editor. J Am Soc Nephrol 1:1260, 1991
19. Cogan MG, Carneiro AV, Tatsumo J et al: Normal diet NaCl variation can affect renal set-point for plasma pH-[HCO_3] maintenance. J Am Soc Nephrol 1:193, 1991
20. Galla JH, Luke RG: Chloride transport and disorders of acid-base balance. Ann Rev Physiol 50:141, 1988
21. Gifford JD, Sharkings K, Work J et al: Total CO_2 transport in rat cortical collecting duct in chloride-depletion alkalosis. Am J Physiol 258:F848, 1990
22. Galla JH, Bonduris DN, Luke RG: Correction of acute chloride-depletion alkalosis in the rat without volume expansion. Am J Physiol 244:F217, 1983
23. Galla JH, Bonduris DN, Luke RG: Effects of chloride and extracellular fluid volume on bicarbonate reabsorption along the nephron in metabolic alkalosis in the rat. J Clin Invest 80:41, 1987
24. Wall BM, Byrum GV, Galla JH, Luke RG: Importance of chloride for the correction of chronic metabolic alkalosis in the rat. Am J Physiol 253:F1031, 1987
25. Xie MH, Liu FY, Cogan MG: Recovery of chronic metabolic alkalosis (CMA). FASEB J 3:A555, 1989
26. Cohen JJ, Ellis JH: Correction of metabolic alkalosis by the kidney after isometric expansion of extracellular fluid. J Clin Invest 47:1181, 1968
27. Liu FY, Cogan M: Role of angiotensin II in glomerulotubular balance. Am J Physiol 259:F72, 1990
28. Kurtzman NA, White MG, Rogers PW: Pathophysiology of metabolic alkalosis. Arch Intern Med 131: 702, 1973
29. Capasso G, Kinne R, Malnic G, Giebisch G: Renal bicarbonate reabsorption in the rat. 1. Effects of hypokalemia and carbonic anhydrase. J Clin Invest 78:1558, 1986
30. Cappasso G, Jaeger P, Giebisch G et al: Renal bicarbonate reabsorption in the rat II. Distal tubule load dependence and effect of hypokalemia. J Clin Invest 80:409, 1987
31. Kassirer JP, Schwartz WB: Correction of metabolic alkalosis in man without repair of potassium deficiency. Am J Med 40:19, 1966
32. Nicolaos M, Adrogue HJ, Cohen JJ: Maladaptive renal response to secondary hypercapnia in chronic metabolic alkalosis. Am J Physiol 238:F283, 1980
33. Berger AJ, Mitchell RA, Severinghaus JW: Medical progress: regulation of respiration. N Engl J Med 297:92, 1977
34. Garella S, Chazan JA, Cohen JJ: Saline-resistant metabolic alkalosis or "chloride-wasting nephropathy." Ann Int Med 73:31, 1970
35. Luke RG, Wright FS, Fowler N et al: Effects of potassium depletion on renal tubular chloride transport in the rat. Kidney Int 14:414, 1978
36. Biglieri EG, Slaton PE, Forsham PH: Useful parameters in the diagnosis of primary aldosteronism. JAMA 178:119, 1961
37. Harrington JT: Metabolic alkalosis. Kidney Int 26:88, 1984
38. Dustan HP, Corcoran AC, Page IH: Renal function in primary aldosteronism. J Clin Invest 35:1357, 1956
39. Milne MD, Muehrcke RC, Aird I: Primary aldosteronism. Quart J Med 26:317, 1957
40. Knepper MA, Packer R, Good DW: Ammonium transport in the kidney. Physiol Rev 69:179, 1989
41. Biglieri EG, Baxter JD: The encocrinology of hypertension. In Felig P, Baxter JD, Broadus AE, Frohrman LA (eds): Endocrinology and Metabolism. McGraw-Hill, New York, 1981
42. Kassirer JP, London AM, Goldman DM, Schwartz WB: On the pathogenesis of metabolic alkalosis in hyperaldosteronism. Am J Med 49:306, 1970
43. Hulter HN, Sigala JF, Sebastian A: K+ deprivation potentiates the renal alkalosis-producing effect of mineralocorticoid. Am J Physiol 235:F298, 1978

7

Mixed Acid-Base Metabolism

George M. Feldman

The use of consistent terminology is important to diagnosing mixed disturbances of acid-base balance, so common terms will be defined at the outset.

Acidemia and alkalemia describe alterations in blood pH.

Acidosis and alkalosis describe processes that shift blood pH in a predictable direction, if nothing intervenes.

Respiratory indicates that the problem is with regulation of PCO_2.

Metabolic indicates that the problem is with regulation of the HCO_3^- concentration.

Compensation refers to secondary changes in PCO_2 or HCO_3^- that result from normal efforts of cells, buffers, lungs, or kidneys to minimize the deviation of pH. In most situations compensation does not bring pH back to normal.

Simple disturbance describes the primary abnormality plus the compensatory changes in PCO_2 and HCO_3^- that result from a single process.

Mixed disturbances are two or more simple disturbances occurring simultaneously. The resulting pH is determined by the relative strengths of the component simple disturbances.

The clinical meaning of the Henderson-Hasselbalch equation is described next.

$$pH = pK + \log \frac{HCO_3^-}{H_2CO_3} = pK + \log \frac{HCO_3^-}{0.03 \times PCO_2} \qquad \text{(Eq. 7-1)}$$

Since pK is constant (6.1), pH is determined by the ratio of

$$\frac{HCO_3^-}{H_2CO_3} \text{ or } \frac{HCO_3^-}{0.03 \times PCO_2}$$

Dedicated to: Bertold Feldman

Table 7-1. Compensation in Disorders of Acid-Base Balance

Metabolic acidosis (>12 h duration)
Expected $PCO_2 = 1.5 \times [HCO_3^-] + 8 \, (\pm 2)$
↓ 1 mEq/L $[HCO_3^-]$
↓ $PCO_2 = 1.25$ mmHg
↓ pH = 0.012 pH unit

Metabolic alkalosis
↑ 1 mEq/L $[HCO_3^-]$
↑ $PCO_2 = 0.7$ mmHg (0.2–0.9 mmHg)
↑ pH = 0.003 to 0.008 pH unit

Respiratory acidosis
Acute
↑ 1 mmHg PCO_2
↑ $[HCO_3^-] = 0.1$ mEq/L
↓ pH = 0.008 pH unit
Chronic (>48 h duration)
↑ 1 mmHg PCO_2
↑ $[HCO_3^-] = 0.5$ mEq/L
↓ pH = 0.0025 pH unit

Respiratory alkalosis
Acute
↓ 1 mmHg = PCO_2
↓ $[HCO_3^-] = 0.25$ mEq/L
↑ pH = 0.007 pH unit
Chronic (>24 h duration)
↓ 1 mmHg PCO_2
↓ $[HCO_3^-] = 0.5$ mEq/L
↓ pH = 0.003 pH unit
After 2 weeks pH may be normal.

The absolute value of HCO_3^- or PCO_2 does not determine pH. Compensation always moves the opposite member of the pair in the same direction to minimize the change in ratio or pH.

Another important concept is that total CO_2 content (tCO_2) is different from HCO_3^-

$$\text{Total } CO_2 = HCO_3^- + (0.03 \times PCO_2) \tag{Eq. 7-2}$$

However, HCO_3^- is the major component of total CO_2. Although both tCO_2 and HCO_3^- concentrations are reported in units of mmol/L or mEq/L, the tCO_2 concentration is typically measured in venous blood, while the HCO_3^- concentration is calculated from the arterial blood pH and PCO_2 (i.e., an ABG). Because venous blood carries metabolically generated CO_2 (in the form of HCO_3^- the tCO_2 concentration (i.e., $[HCO_3^-] + [CO_2]$) in venous blood is generally 2 to 5 mmol/L greater than the HCO_3^- concentration in arterial blood.*

Impractical ways of recognizing a mixed acid-base disturbances include: (1) memorize all compensatory changes (Table 7-1). (2) carry an acid-base nomogram.[3,4] It may confirm a sus-

---

* Additional discrepancies between tCO_2 and HCO_3^- values occur occasionally and are thought to result from variations in the pK (an assumed constant in the Henderson-Hasselbalch equation) used to calculate HCO_3^-. Unfortunately, studies reporting these discrepancies failed to assess the accuracy of the pH, PCO_2 and tCO_2 measurements, and it is likely that the errors in these measurements, especially in the determination of PCO_2 and tCO_2, account for the unexpected discrepancies between tCO_2 and HCO_3^-.[1,2]

pected mixed disturbance. (3) Neither a nomogram nor application of compensatory changes exclude a mixed acid-base disturbance. Therefore, these tools should be used as a check, not as means of making a diagnosis.

It is important to know a few generalities, such as, compensation never overshoots. Also, compensation rarely brings the pH back to the normal pH range (remember the width of the normal range). The only common exception is chronic respiratory alkalosis. The following are true: (1) in pure respiratory alkalosis, HCO_3^- is never below 10; (2) in pure metabolic alkalosis, PCO_2 is rarely above 60; and (3) in pure *metabolic acidosis,* Winters' formula predicts the PCO_2.[5]

$$PCO_2 = 1.5 \times HCO_3^- + 8 \ (\pm 2)$$ (Eq. 7-3)

Values beyond these limits strongly suggest a mixed disturbance. Because Winters' formula was derived from ABG values, the arterial HCO_3^- concentration should be used to calculate the expected PCO_2 compared to the measured PCO_2.

Finally, don't overdiagnose mixed disturbances, especially in a rapidly changing situation (e.g., the recovery phase of any simple disturbance), because compensation lags. For example, in rapidly correcting diabetic ketoacidosis, respiratory compensation persists despite improving metabolism, giving the appearance of respiratory alkalosis plus metabolic acidosis. In other words, acid-base disturbances result from dynamic processes, and a single (static) ABG determination does not necessarily represent the clinical situation.

The best method is to use to diagnose a mixed acid-base disturbance is a systematic approach (Fig. 7-1).[6]

First, use the history; consider symptoms. For example, *vomiting* usually causes metabolic alkalosis; *diarrhea* usually causes metabolic acidosis; *dyspnea* suggests respiratory alkalosis, but when severe, respiratory acidosis can occur; and *polyuria* is frequently present in diabetic ketoacidosis.

Second, consider disease states. For example, *congestive heart failure* alters ventilation/perfusion in the lung and induces respiratory alkalosis[7,8]; *diabetes mellitus* can cause metabolic (keto-) acidosis; *chronic obstructive pulmonary disease* causes respiratory acidosis; and *liver disease* can be associated with respiratory alkalosis.[9,10]

Third, consider medications. For example, *sedatives* can cause respiratory acidosis; *diuretics* typically cause metabolic alkalosis, except carbonic anhydrase inhibitors (e.g., acetazolamide), which cause metabolic acidosis; and *laxatives* can cause metabolic acidosis.

Consider past or current treatments. For example, *mechanical ventilation* can cause either respiratory acidosis or respiratory alkalosis, depending on machine settings; *nasogastric suction* causes metabolic alkalosis[11]; and *intravenous fluids* can contain H^+ or HCO_3^- (e.g., HCl, arginine-HCl, $NaHCO_3$, sodium lactate).

Next, use the physical examination: *tetany* suggests metabolic or respiratory alkalosis, because alkalemia increases binding of Ca^{2+} to albumin, consequently decreasing the ionized Ca^{2+} concentration; *jaundice* suggests respiratory alkalosis (elevated NH_3 levels and unmetabolized toxins in liver disease induce hyperventilation); *cyanosis* suggests respiratory acidosis (decreased ventilation); and *Kussmaul breathing* (deep, regular respirations) suggests acidemia due to metabolic acidosis.

Finally, examine the laboratory data; they provide important clues to the patient's status. Routine laboratory data can indicate such things as renal disease, liver disease, or sepsis. Key data to obtain are electrolytes and blood gases. If tCO_2 is abnormal, there must be at least a single disturbance; if it is normal, there may be multiple disturbances.

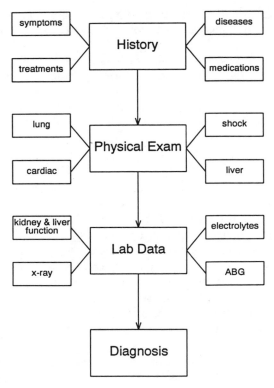

Fig. 7-1. Schematic approach to the evaluation of mixed acid-base disorders.

The anion gap is determined by the following equation[12,13]

$$Na^+ - (tCO_2 + Cl^-) \qquad \text{(Eq. 7-4)}$$

If the result is greater than 16, then metabolic acidosis is likely (or lab error). A normal AG, however, does not exclude metabolic acidosis. Because albumin has a net negative charge, albumin contributes significantly to the normal AG (3 to 12 mEq/L); other important unmeasured anions also contribute to the AG, including phosphate, urate, lactate, and sulfate. Besides laboratory errors, the calculated AG is affected by a variety of factors. Hypoalbuminemia reduces the AG. Acidemia reduces albumin's electronegativity and consequently reduces the AG, while alkalemia increases the AG.[14,15] Elevated Ca^{2+}, Mg^{2+} and Li^+ concentrations, or the presence of Br^-, which falsely elevates the Cl^- concentration, reduce the AG.[16,17] Multiple myeloma producing excess cationic γ-globulins reduces the AG or can cause a negative AG.[18,19] High carbenicillin concentrations, especially in renal failure, and excess anionic γ-globulins increase the AG. Because newer laboratory techniques yield different Cl^- and tCO_2 values, the AG is altered unpredictably, especially in very ill patients.[2,20–23]

In uncomplicated AG acidosis, the increase in the AG (Δ AG) should equal the decrease in the tCO_2 concentration (ΔtCO_2). A difference in these two values is called the delta (Δ) gap.[24] For example, a 5 mEq/L rise in the AG (Δ AG) should result in a 5 mEq/L fall in the tCO_2

concentration (Δ tCO_2). A significant deviation in stoichiometry implies a mixed acid-base disorder. The calculation of Δ gap follows.

$$\Delta \text{ gap} = \Delta \text{ AG} - \Delta \text{ tCO}_2 \text{ (range } \pm 6 \text{ mEq/L)}$$
$$\Delta \text{ AG} = \text{observed AG} - 12 \qquad \qquad \text{(Eq. 7-5)}$$
$$\Delta \text{ tCO}_2 = 28 - \text{observed tCO}_2$$

This calculation has utility when evaluating the possibility of simultaneous widened anion gap type metabolic acidosis and metabolic alkalosis. Under these conditions, the Δ Gap will be positive, because the Δ AG (i.e., widening of the AG) is greater than the Δ tCO_2 (i.e., the acidosis-induced decrement in the $[tCO_2]$ will be offset by the increment in $[tCO_2]$ due to the metabolic alkalosis). All the limitations of the AG apply to the Δ gap. Moreover, the Δ gap is not universally accepted and has not been applied to large numbers of patients.

Serum K gives a clue to metabolic disorders, because the K concentration may predict the direction of the pH change. However, remember that the serum K concentration is regulated independently.

Blood gases should be measured when the above steps suggest a mixed acid-base disturbance or a grossly abnormal pH. The following list ranks blood gas measurements by their importance to a diagnosis.

Arterial blood gas (ABG): The best. In addition to pH and PCO_2, the PO_2 is invaluable in a serious clinical situation.

Arteriolized venous: The next best in adults and easiest to obtain in children.

Venous, peripheral: This is poor, because it will not reflect systemic picture accurately and PO_2 is useless.

Venous, central (i.e., right heart or pulmonary artery): Obtained infrequently, a central venous blood gas is helpful in assessing cardiac function. Central venous blood is the effluent of metabolizing tissues. Because tissues extract O_2 and add CO_2 at a fairly constant rate, the amount of O_2 extracted from and CO_2 added to a given volume of blood will vary inversely with blood flow. Therefore, the central venous PO_2, PCO_2 and pH values will be influenced by cardiac output, and the most obvious effect will be when cardiac output is reduced: $\downarrow$ CO $\rightarrow$ $\downarrow$ PO_2, $\uparrow$ PCO_2 and $\downarrow$ pH. At the same time arterial blood values will reflect the efficacy of ventilation and will likely show $\uparrow$ PO_2 and $\downarrow$ PCO_2.[25]

Two questions guide your interpretation of ABG: Are they consistent with your diagnosis? From a nomogram are they possible? Use the PO_2 to calculate the Alveolar-arteriolar (A-a) O_2 gradient ($PaO_2 - PaO_2$). The alveolar PO_2 is calculated as

$$PaO_2 = PiO_2 - \frac{PCO_2}{R.Q.} = 150 - \frac{PCO_2}{0.8} = 150 - (1.25 \times PCO_2) \qquad \text{(Eq. 7-6)}$$

where PiO_2 is the inspired O_2 tension and R.Q. is the respiratory quotient. An increased A-a gradient indicates a ventilation-perfusion defect or shunting blood flow. It may be the first sign of impending respiratory failure or pulmonary emboli. Breathing room air at sea level, the normal A-a gradient is less than 10 mmHg in young people and increases with age, but should not exceed 25 mmHg in people older than 65 years.

GENERAL READINGS

Alpern RJ, Stone DK, Rector FC Jr: Renal acidification mechanisms. p. 318. In Brenner BM, Rector FC Jr (eds): The Kidney. 4th Ed. WB Saunders, Philadelphia, 1991

Cogan MG, Rector FC Jr: Acid-Base disorders. p. 737. In Brenner BM, Rector FC Jr (eds): The Kidney. 4th Ed. WB Saunders, Philadelphia, 1991

Davenport HW: The ABC's of Acid-Base Chemistry. 6th Ed. University of Chicago Press, Chicago, 1974
Emmett M, Narins RG: Clinical use of the anion gap. Medicine 56:38, 1977
Madias NE: Lactic acidosis. Kidney Int 29:752, 1986

CASE STUDY 1

Ms. Linda Blake, a 32-year-old woman with chronic pyelonephritis associated with a congenital urethral anomaly, had been relatively asymptomatic on a high fluid, low protein regimen. Over the past 6 weeks she developed weakness, nausea, occasional vomiting and exertional dyspnea. These symptoms became progressively more severe, so she was admitted to the hospital. At admission her physical examination revealed a blood pressure of 160/100, neck vein distention, a S_3 gallop, dullness to percussion at the base of both lungs, bilateral crepitant rales, and moderate tachypnea. She did not have peripheral edema. Chest x-ray revealed increased pulmonary vasculature and bilateral large pleural effusions. Blood studies were obtained.

Three hours after admission an attempt was made to remove the pleural effusion, but the tap was unsuccessful. Within minutes, her dyspnea increased markedly following which she arrested as another set of blood studies were drawn. She responded to intubation and placement of a chest tube.

LABORATORY DATA

Blood Studies

	BUN (mg/dL)	Cr* (mg/dL)	Na (mEq/L)	K (mEq/L)	Cl (mEq/L)	tCO₂	Arterial pH	Arterial PCO₂	Arterial HCO₃⁻ (mEq/L)
admission	175	18	130	5.0	90	18	7.40	26	16
3 hours later	180	18.4	131	5.2	88	11	6.90	50	9.3

* Creatinine

Question 1. **Does the history suggest the existence of acid-base disorders? Which disorders are possible?**

Question 2. **Does the physical examination suggest the existence of acid-base disorders? Which disorders are possible?**

Question 3. **Does the laboratory data indicate the existence of acid-base disorders? Which disorders are possible?**

Question 4. **After integrating the information from the history, physical examination and laboratory data, which acid-base disorders does this patient have?**

Question 5. **How would you treat this patient?**

1. Does the history suggest the existence of acid-base disorders? Which disorders are possible?

The patient's history of "chronic pyelonephritis" indicates longstanding renal disease, and her symptoms of weakness, nausea, and vomiting are consistent with renal failure. When the GFR is sufficiently reduced (<15 to 20 mL/min) unmeasured anions are retained and the anion gap is increased.[26] Her symptom of exertional dyspnea probably relates to fluid retention that results from renal failure rather than primary heart disease, and increased pulmonary fluid is a potent stimulus of ventilation, which could induce respiratory alkalosis as long as pulmonary gas exchange is not compromised. Although vomiting can induce metabolic alkalosis, the infrequency of vomiting episodes is unlikely to have a large impact on acid-base balance.

Events in the hospital could also contribute to an acid-base disturbance. The unsuccessful thoracentesis was followed by sudden worsening of the patient's dyspnea, suggesting the development of a pneumothorax. A pneumothorax would compromise the ventilatory ability and cause respiratory acidosis as well as hypoxemia. The latter will induce lactic acidosis.

2. Does the physical examination suggest the existence of acid-base disorders? Which disorders are possible?

The patient's physical examination (modest elevation of blood pressure, distended neck vein, and S_3 gallop) is entirely consistent with a congested circulatory system due to volume overload. The physical findings also revealed a pleural effusion that was accompanied with tachypnea, supporting the possibility of respiratory alkalosis.

3. Does the laboratory data indicate the existence of acid-base disorders? Which disorders are possible?

Her chest x-ray showed a large effusion, which raises the possibility of respiratory alkalosis. The initial blood studies revealed marked elevations of BUN and creatinine, indicating renal failure. The obvious reduction in tCO_2 suggests metabolic acidosis consistent with renal failure and the widened anion gap of 22 (AG = Na^+ of 130 − (Cl^- of 90 + tCO_2 of 18)) is also consistent with renal failure. The initial ABG showed a normal pH, but both HCO_3^- and PCO_2 were low. To assess whether metabolic acidosis (i.e., the primary disturbance with respiratory compensation) could account for the ABG results, Winters' formula can be applied (expected $PCO_2 = 1.5 \times [HCO_3^-] + 8 (\pm 2)$). However, because the predicted PCO_2 is 32 mmHg and higher than the observed PCO_2 of 26 mmHg, metabolic acidosis could not account for her respiratory status, raising the possibility of combined disorders: metabolic acidosis and respiratory alkalosis.

During the patient's cardiorespiratory arrest, the serum tCO_2 decreased further and the anion gap widened to 32. This pattern is consistent with the development of lactic acidosis due to hypoxemia and cardiovascular collapse. The simultaneous ABG revealed a very low pH, elevated PCO_2 and depressed HCO_3^- This pattern is consistent with the patient's initial problem of metabolic acidosis due renal failure and the subsequent acute problems of lactic acidosis and hypoventilation due to cardiopulmonary arrest.

4. After integrating the information from the history, physical examination, and laboratory data, which acid-base disorders does this patient have?

This patient's mixed acid-base disturbances are easily identified if the clinical information is interpreted prior to assessing the laboratory data. Initially, she was admitted with metabolic acidosis due to renal failure and respiratory alkalosis due to fluid overload–induced pleural effusions. In the hospital, ventilatory failure induced by lactic acidosis occurred, worsening her metabolic acidosis and acute respiratory acidosis.

5. How would you treat this patient?

The patient's most urgent problem was ventilatory failure due to the pneumothorax, and this was correctly treated with a chest tube. As a result, her electrolytes and ABG quickly returned to her admission values. The remaining therapy was directed at her underlying problem, renal failure, and hemodialysis was initiated. With dialysis her volume overload state and her metabolic acidosis were corrected. After several treatments, her pleural effusion disappeared and she began routine thrice weekly dialytic treatment. She also decided to undergo renal transplantation and her name was placed on the transplant list.

CASE STUDY 2

Mr. Mel Smith, a 71-year-old retired storekeeper, was admitted to the hospital for evaluation of anemia, and blood studies were obtained. On evaluation he was found to have carcinoma of the transverse colon, and the lesion was surgically resected. Postoperative 24-hour urine volumes were 800 to 1200 mL, and nasogastric drainage averaged 1500 mL each day. On the fifth postoperative day, his temperature rose to 102.6°F, but his blood pressure was unchanged. Physical examination suggested basilar pneumonitis, and the area around the wound was indurated. An intra-abdominal abscess was also suspected. Blood cultures were drawn and he was started on antibiotics. All cultures were positive for *Pseudomonas* species. Additional blood studies were obtained on the sixth postoperative day. The exact composition of the intake fluid was not clear from the chart, but the administered volume appeared to equal measured losses plus 500 mL/day.

LABORATORY DATA

Blood Studies

	BUN (mg/dL)	Cr* (mg/dL)	Na (mEq/L)	K (mEq/L)	Cl (mEq/L)	tCO_2	Arterial pH	Arterial PCO_2	Arterial HCO_3^- (mEq/L)
admission	11	1.2	140	4.3	100	27	—	—	—
day 6	88	8.1	140	4.2	90	24	7.43	32	21

Question 1. Does the history suggest the existence of acid-base disorders? Which disorders are possible?

Question 2. Does the physical examination suggest the existence of acid-base disorders? Which disorders are possible?

Question 3. Does the laboratory data indicate the existence of acid-base disorders? Which disorders are possible?

Question 4. After integrating the information from the history, physical examination and laboratory data, which acid-base disorders does this patient have?

Question 5. How would you treat this patient?

1. Does the history suggest the existence of acid-base disorders? Which disorders are possible?

The patient's hospital course suggests multiple possible disturbances of acid-base balance. In this elderly man, a surgical complication, such as hypotension, could lead to acute renal failure and consequently metabolic acidosis. During the postoperative period nasogastric suction can cause metabolic alkalosis,[27] while gram negative sepsis can lead to acute renal failure and consequent metabolic acidosis, even without hypotension or shock. Of course, sepsis-induced hypotension is a cause of lactic acidosis.

2. Does the physical examination suggest the existence of acid-base disorders? Which disorders are possible?

On the fifth hospital day, the physical findings of fever, pneumonia, an indurated wound, and possible intra-abdominal abscess are also suggestive of acid-base disturbances. Pneumonia early in its course (before ventilatory failure) can induce respiratory alkalosis, while lactic acidosis can be a consequence of a severe infection that causes hypotension. Because the patient was not hypotensive, lactic acidosis is unlikely.

3. Does the laboratory data indicate the existence of acid-base disorders? Which disorders are possible?

Initial blood studies showed normal acid-base balance. Blood cultures taken on the fifth day were positive for *Pseudomonas* species, indicating sepsis, which could cause hypotension and consequently lactic acidosis. On the sixth postoperative day, the elevated BUN and creatinine concentrations indicate renal failure and suggest that metabolic acidosis is likely. Indeed, the widening of the AG from an upper limit of 12 to the value of 26 is consistent with metabolic acidosis due to renal failure, but the tCO_2 is only minimally depressed. That is, the stoichiometry 1 mEq of H^+ for each mEq increase in AG means that the widening of the AG (or Δ AG) of 14 represents a release of 14 mEq/L of H^+, which should have reduced the tCO_2 from 27 to 13 mEq/L. The lack of fall in tCO_2 concentration reveals the existence of metabolic alkalosis. The Δ gap of 11 mEq/L reveals the same information: Δ gap $= \Delta$ AG of 14 $- \Delta tCO_2$ (or fall in tCO_2) of 3. Meanwhile, the ABG revealed a normal pH, low PCO_2 and low HCO_3^-; the low PCO_2 without acidemia suggests respiratory alkalosis.

4. After integrating information from the history, physical examination, and laboratory data, which acid-base disorders does this patient have?

In this case renal failure probably occurred at the time of surgery, as evidenced by the elevated BUN and creatinine 6 days after surgery. In the absence of rhabdomyolosis and rapid leak of creatinine from muscle, acute renal failure causes the serum creatinine to rise at a maximal rate of 1 to 2 mg/dL per day. Over the 6-day interval following surgery, metabolically produced acids would be retained, causing a metabolic acidosis and widened anion gap. The lack of reduction in tCO_2 is accounted for by nasogastric suction and consequent metabolic alkalosis. Thus, metabolic acidosis is neutralized by metabolic alkalosis. In addition, the ABG reveals a mild degree of respiratory alkalosis due to pneumonia.

5. How would you treat this patient?

Therapy should be directed at the underlying problem, namely infection(s). Although antibiotic therapy may be sufficient, the possibility of an intra-abdominal abscess must be investigated vigorously and surgery may be necessary. Hemodialysis is indicated if renal function does not improve in the next several days.

CASE STUDY 3

Mr. L. Bobender, a 44-year-old patient with known chronic alcoholism, came to the emergency room. He was obviously intoxicated, but also complained of severe abdominal pain that radiated to his back, nausea, vomiting, and dyspnea. Physical examination showed a blood pressure of 110/60 mmHg, pulse of 115 and respiratory rate of 28 per min. His abdomen was rigid with diffuse tenderness and hypoactive bowel sounds. There was dullness to percussion at the right base of his chest. The patient's visual acuity and visual fields appeared to be intact and retinal exam revealed normal eye grounds. On chest x-ray, a large effusion and consolidation was present in the right base.

LABORATORY DATA

Blood Studies

	BUN (mg/dL)	Cr (mg/dL)	Na (mEq/L)	K (mEq/L)	Cl (mEq/L)	tCO_2	Arterial pH	Arterial PCO_2	Arterial PO_2	HCO_3^- (mEq/L)
admission	47	1.6	142	3.4	92	22	7.28	41	58	19

Additional Studies

Blood			Urine	
amylase (IU)	glucose (mg/dL)	ketones	ketones	crystals
915	150	1+	4+	None

Question 1. Does the history suggest the existence of acid-base disorders? Which disorders are possible?

Question 2. Does the physical examination suggest the existence of acid-base disorders? Which disorders are possible?

Question 3. **Does the laboratory data indicate the existence of acid-base disorders? Which disorders are possible?**

Question 4. **After integrating the information from the history, physical examination and laboratory data, which acid-base disorders does this patient have?**

Question 5. **How would you treat this patient?**

---

1. Does the history suggest the existence of acid-base disorders? Which disorders are possible?

Acute ethanol intoxication, especially when characterized by binge drinking, no food intake, vomiting, and abdominal pain, suggests alcoholic ketoacidosis.[28] At the cellular level, it is thought that the combination of starvation and ethanol intake alters the redox potential, resulting in increased serum levels of various organic acids, including β-hydroxy-butyric, lactic, and free fatty acids. Consideration should also be given to the ingestion of alternate alcohols such as methanol and ethylene glycol. In addition to the above possibilities, the history of severe abdominal pain and vomiting is consistent with gastritis, peptic ulcer disease, and/or acute pancreatitis. Alcoholic ketoacidosis is a form of anion gap metabolic acidosis, and pancreatitis can also cause a widened anion gap acidosis (lactic acidosis). Vomiting, of course, will induce metabolic alkalosis, and vomiting in an intoxicated person can lead to aspiration and pneumonia. Dyspnea, if accompanied with increased ventilation, will lead to respiratory alkalosis, but if ventilation is compromised respiratory acidosis will follow.

2. Does the physical examination suggest the existence of acid-base disorders? Which disorders are possible?

On physical examination, tachycardia and a borderline low blood pressure are suggestive of decreased ECF volume status. A tender abdomen and hypoactive bowel sounds are consistent with acute abdominal processes, including peptic ulcer disease, gastritis, and acute pancreatitis. Tachypnea and dullness to percussion at the base of his chest are consistent with a significant pleural effusion and/or pneumonia, impairing ventilation. Intact visual fields and normal retinal exam suggest that methanol had not been ingested, but are not definitive.

3. Does the laboratory data indicate the existence of acid-base disorders? Which disorders are possible?

The large effusion and consolidation on chest x-ray are consistent with impaired pulmonary function, possibly leading to respiratory acidosis. Serum electrolytes reveal a mildly decreased tCO_2 concentration and an increased anion gap, suggesting metabolic acidosis. Calculation of the Δ gap yields a value of 10 (i.e., Δ Gap $=$ Δ AG or $[28 - 12] - \Delta tCO_2$ or $[28 - 22]$), suggesting that metabolic alkalosis is also present. Interestingly, low K^+ concentration is also consistent with metabolic alkalosis. The near normal renal function, as indicated by the near normal creatinine, does not explain the widened anion gap. The ABG reveals acidemia and a low HCO_3^-, which are consistent with metabolic acidosis. However, the observed PCO_2 of 41 is elevated as compared to the expected PCO_2 of 36 (Winters' formula; expected $PCO_2 = 1.5 \times [HCO_3^-] + 8 \ (\pm 2)$), demonstrating respiratory acidosis.

Additional blood studies revealed an elevated amylase consistent with pancreatitis. The elevated serum and urine ketone by nitroprusside indicates an elevated acetoacetate level, but the minimally elevated glucose concentration suggests starvation or alcoholic ketoacidosis as the etiology, not diabetic ketoacidosis. Because ketone bodies are filtered and not reabsorbed by the kidney, urine ketone concentrations are significantly higher than serum values in starvation and alcoholic ketoacidosis. However, if ketones are produced at a prodigious rate as in diabetic ketoacidosis, serum ketones can be quite elevated. Absence of crystals (i.e., oxalate and hippurate crystals) in the urine indicates that ethylene glycol had not been ingested.

4. After integrating the information from the history, physical examination, and laboratory data, which acid-base disorders does this patient have?

Considering the patient's intoxication, vomiting, and mildly positive serum ketones, the widened anion gap acidosis presumably represents alcoholic ketoacidosis, but pancreatitis is certainly present and is a cause of lactic acidosis. In addition, vomiting-induced metabolic alkalosis minimized the reduction in bicarbonate concentration caused by metabolic acidosis. Impaired ventilation prevented the appropriate respiratory compensation for metabolic acidosis and resulted in respiratory acidosis.

It is also important to consider methanol intoxication, and to send a blood sample for analysis, despite an apparently normal ophthamologic examination. This evaluation may be aided by calculating the osmolal gap (the difference between the measured osmolality and the calculated osmolality).* If the osmolal gap is small (<10) then the serum does not contain an unmeasured solute, such as ethanol or methanol. If, however, the osmolal gap is significant, an unmeasured solute is present. The contribution of ethanol to the osmolal gap can be estimated from the ethanol level and ethanol's formula weight of 46. If reported in units of mg/dL, divide by 4.6 to obtain the osmolality units of mOsm/kg.

5. How would you treat this patient?

The treatment of this patient should be directed at the following problems: pneumonia and consequent ventilatory compromise, borderline hemodynamic status, pancreatitis and alcoholic ketoacidosis. Administration of antibiotics, supplemental O_2, possible intubation and ventilatory support, sputum gram stain and culture, as well as thoracentesis are all appropriate to manage the patient's pulmonary condition. Intravenous fluids, specifically normal saline, should be administered in order to replete the patient's ECF volume. Nasogastric suction is a reasonable first step to evaluate the patient's abdominal pain. This supportive care, plus the addition of glucose to the administered intravenous fluids, should be a sufficient first step in treating the starvation component of alcoholic ketoacidosis, and time will permit ethanol to be fully metabolized. Frequent monitoring of the serum K^+ and phosphate levels are indicated, because in situations of refeeding following starvation, hypokalemia and hypophosphatemia can occur. These deficiency states require vigorous supplementation in order to avoid rhabdomyolysis.

CASE STUDY 4

Mr. Blackie Hill, a 53-year-old coal miner, had a chronic cough and dyspnea on exertion for a number of years. On a visit to his daughter, he caught a "cold" and over the next 3 days developed a marked increase in his sputum production, dyspnea, fever, and confusion. On admission he

---

* Calculated osmolality $= 2 \times Na^+ + \dfrac{glucose}{18} + \dfrac{BUN}{2.8}$

was febrile (102°F), cyanotic and semistuporous, and had a physical examination that was characteristic of chronic emphysema, including a widened AP diameter, hyper-resonance, and decreased breath sounds. He was intubated, placed on a respiratory, and given 5% dextrose in 0.5 normal saline (77 mEq/L NaCl) intravenously. Potassium chloride and antibiotics were also administered intravenously, and bronchodialator therapy was initiated.

LABORATORY DATA

Blood Studies

	BUN (mg/ dL)	Cr (mg/ dL)	Na (mEq/ L)	K (mEq/ L)	Cl (mEq/ L)	tCO_2	pH	Arterial PCO_2	HCO_3^- (mEq/ L)
admission	14	1.2	140	4.9	84	45	7.18	96	35
next day	14	1.2	139	4.1	92	34	7.48	39	29

Question 1. Does the history suggest the existence of acid-base disorders? Which disorders are possible?

Question 2. Does the physical examination suggest the existence of acid-base disorders? Which disorders are possible?

Question 3. Does the laboratory data indicate the existence of acid-base disorders? Which disorders are possible?

Question 4. After integrating the information from the history, physical examination and laboratory data, which acid-base disorders does this patient have?

Question 5. How would you treat this patient?

---

1. Does the history suggest the existence of acid-base disorders? Which disorders are possible?

This man has a history consistent with chronic obstructive pulmonary disease. Thus, it would not be surprising if he had chronic respiratory acidosis and if his baseline ABG revealed acidemia, an elevated PCO_2, and an elevated HCO_3^- The patient developed a "cold" and worsening symptoms, cough, sputum production, and dyspnea. The addition of fever to his symptoms suggests pneumonia and thus increased CO_2 retention is expected. Once in the hospital, intubation and ventilator assistance allow therapeutic manipulation of the respiratory component of acid-base balance.

2. Does the physical examination suggest the existence of acid-base disorders? Which disorders are possible?

The chest findings of increased AP diameter, hyper-resonance, and decreased breath sounds are entirely consistent with COPD, while cyanosis and semi-stupor indicate hypoxemia and CO_2 retention to the point of CO_2 narcosis.

3. Does the laboratory data indicate the existence of acid-base disorders? Which disorders are possible?

Serum electrolytes on admission revealed an elevated tCO_2, depressed Cl^-, and normal anion gap, all consistent with chronic respiratory acidosis or primary metabolic alkalosis. The ABG showed a markedly elevated PCO_2 and acidemia, suggesting respiratory acidosis. In chronic respiratory acidosis, the pH is reduced 0.0025 pH unit for each 1 mmHg elevation in PCO_2. Therefore, if this patient had chronic respiratory acidosis, his 56 mmHg increment in PCO_2 indicates that the pH should be 7.26. Because his measured pH is more acid than that expected for chronic respiratory acidosis, an additional form of acidosis exists, either metabolic or acute respiratory. Since the PCO_2 is remarkably elevated, beyond that commonly seen in chronic respiratory acidosis, acute respiratory acidosis is likely.

Following less than 1 day of treatment in the hospital, repeat blood studies revealed slightly altered electrolytes, but remarkably different ABG values, a normal PCO_2, alkaline pH and elevated HCO_3^-. These values are more consistent with metabolic alkalosis than respiratory acidosis. However, in metabolic alkalosis one would expect the PCO_2 to be about 43 (i.e., ~0.7 mmHg rise in PCO_2 for each mEq/L rise in HCO_3^-) rather than the observed value of 39 mmHg.

4. After integrating the information from the history, physical examination, and laboratory data, which acid-base disorders does this patient have?

The patient's history suggests that he had both chronic respiratory acidosis and superimposed acute respiratory acidosis, and these diagnoses were supported by his admitting blood studies. Less than 1 day after initiating ventilator assistance, the patient's PCO_2 was 39 mmHg and he had metabolic alkalosis. In chronic respiratory acidosis, the HCO_3^- generated in compensation for CO_2 retention must be excreted by the kidneys following improved ventilation. Although the kidneys can readily excrete excess HCO_3^-, when a patient is volume and/or Cl^- depleted, renal HCO_3^- excretion is impaired by increased tubular HCO_3^- reabsorption.[27] Frequently, patients with chronic respiratory acidosis are treated with a low-salt diet and diuretics, and consequently they are Cl^- depleted. This Cl^- deficiency is not manifest until ventilation is improved and hypercapnia is corrected.[29,30] At that point the lack of renal HCO_3^- excretion manifests itself as posthypercapneic metabolic alkalosis.[30]

5. How would you treat this patient?

Therapy for this patient should first be directed at his acute and chronic pulmonary problems as was done. Treatment of posthypercapneic metabolic alkalosis simply requires NaCl, and this can be administered either orally or intravenously.

CASE STUDY 5

Ms. Sally, a 66-year-old woman, had a long history of both Laennec's cirrhosis and chronic glomerulonephritis. She had been asymptomatic for the past year on a regimen of salt restriction and a low-protein diet. Recently, however, abdominal distension and dependent edema had been a problem in spite of treatment with hydrochlorthiazide and spironolactone. Increasing irritability, confusion, and weight gain finally prompted admission. She was tremulous and mildly icteric with a blood pressure of 150/90, respiratory rate of 22 and pulse of 88. Other positive findings included spider nevi, marked abdominal distention with shifting dullness, elevated diaphragms with bilateral basilar rales, and 1+ ankle edema. The liver could not be palpated. There was a course flapping tremor of the outstretched hands.

LABORATORY DATA

Blood Studies

| | BUN (mg/ dL) | Cr (mg/ dL) | Na (mEq/ L) | K (mEq/ L) | Cl (mEq/ L) | tCO$_2$ | Arterial | | |
							pH	PCO$_2$	HCO$_3^-$ (mEq/ L)
admission	58	7.2	135	4.0	96	17	7.47	21	15

Question 1. Does the history suggest the existence of acid-base disorders? Which disorders are possible?

Question 2. Does the physical examination suggest the existence of acid-base disorders? Which disorders are possible?

Question 3. Does the laboratory data indicate the existence of acid-base disorders? Which disorders are possible?

Question 4. After integrating the information from the history, physical examination and laboratory data, which acid-base disorders does this patient have?

Question 5. How would you treat this patient?

1. Does the history suggest the existence of acid-base disorders? Which disorders are possible?

Cirrhosis causes hyperventilation and consequently respiratory alkalosis, but the mechanism is unknown.[9,10,31] Renal failure is an obvious cause of metabolic acidosis. In patients with normal renal function, hydrochlorthiazide and spironolactone have opposing effects on acid-base balance. Hydrochlorthiazide can induce metabolic alkalosis.[32] Because hydrochlorthiazide causes volume depletion, angiotensin II levels are increased. AII stimulates proximal tubule reabsorption of HCO$_3^-$ and adrenal production of aldosterone. Hyperaldosteronism augments tubular secretion of K$^+$ and H$^+$, and the resulting K$^+$ depletion increases ammonia synthesis and urinary NH$_4^+$ excretion. Thus, hydrochlorthiazide stimulates net acid excretion (i.e., generation of a base load) and renal HCO$_3^-$ reabsorption (i.e., maintenance of the elevated HCO$_3^-$). In contrast, spironolactone, an inhibitor of aldosterone, reduces K^+ and H^+ secretion and, thus, blunts some of the hydrochlorthiazide effects.

2. Does the physical examination suggest the existence of acid-base disorders? Which disorders are possible?

The patient's physical findings of elevated BP, ascites, and peripheral edema demonstrate increased extracellular volume, and the presence of ascites, icterus, and spider nevi demonstrate impaired liver function. An altered mental state and course flapping tremor of outstretched hands, asterixis, can occur in endstage renal disease or liver disease.

3. Does the laboratory data indicate the existence of acid-base disorders? Which disorders are possible?

The elevated BUN and creatinine demonstrate kidney failure, and the low tCO_2 and widened anion gap are consistent with metabolic acidosis due to renal failure. However, the ABG reveals alkalemia and a remarkably decreased PCO_2, consistent with respiratory alkalosis.

4. After integrating the information from the history, physical examination, and laboratory data, which acid-base disorders does this patient have?

Metabolic acidosis due to renal failure and respiratory alkalosis due to liver failure are both present in this very ill woman. For diuretics to be effective there must be sufficient renal mass and a sufficient number of functioning tubules to respond to these agents. Since the patient has little renal function remaining, the diuretics have little effect (note the patient's anasarca in the face of diuretic usage) and are not a cause of metabolic alkalosis.

5. How would you treat this patient?

Therapy for this patient should be directed at her liver failure and renal failure. Although hemodialysis can effectively replace renal function, this patient's profound liver disease cannot be treated. Therefore, hemodialysis is not an indicated therapy.

REFERENCES

1. Rivkees SA, Fine BP: The reliability of calculated bicarbonate in clinical practice. Clin Pediatr 27:240, 1988
2. Mohler JG, Mohler PA, Pallivathucal RG: Failure of the serum CO_2 determined by automation to estimate the plasma bicarbonate. Scand J Clin Lab Invest Suppl 188:61, 1987
3. Goldberg M, Green SB, Moss ML et al: Computer-based instruction and diagnosis of acid-base disorders: a systematic approach. JAMA 233:269, 1973
4. Cogan MG, Rector JC Jr: Acid-Base Disorders. p. 737. In Brenner BM, Rector FC Jr (eds): The Kidney. 4th Ed. WB Saunders, Philadelphia, 1991
5. Albert MS, Dell RB, Winters RW: Quantitative displacement of acid-base equilibrium in metabolic acidosis. Ann Intern Med 66:313, 1967
6. McCurdy DK: Mixed metabolic and respiratory acid-base disturbances: diagnosis and treatment. Chest 62:35S, 1972
7. Buller NP, Poole Wilson PA: Mechanism of the increased ventilatory response to exercise in patients with chronic heart failure. Br Heart J 63:281, 1990
8. Poole Wilson PA, Buller NP: Causes of symptoms in chronic congestive heart failure and implications for treatment. Am J Cardiol 62:31A, 1988

9. Agusti AG, Roca J, Rodriguez Roisin R et al: Pulmonary hemodynamics and gas exchange during exercise in liver cirrhosis. Am Rev Respir Dis 139:485, 1989
10. Oster JR, Perez GO: Acid-base disturbances in liver disease. J Hepatol 2:299, 1986
11. Seldin DW, Rector FC Jr: the generation and maintenance of metabolic alkalosis. Kidney Int 1:306, 1972
12. Emmett M, Narins RG: Clinical use of the anion gap. Medicine 56:38, 1977
13. Oh MS, Carroll HJ: The anion gap. N Engl J Med 297:814, 1977
14. Madias NE, Ayus JC, Adrogue HJ: Increased anion gap in metabolic alkalosis. The role of plasma-protein equivalency. N Engl J Med 300:1421, 1979
15. Adrogue HJ, Brensilver J, Madias NE: Changes in plasma anion gap during chronic metabolic acid-base disturbances. Am J Physiol 235:F291, 1978
16. Kelleher SP, Raciti A, Arbeit LA: Reduced or absent serum anion gap as a marker of severe lithium intoxication. Arch Intern Med 146:1839, 1986
17. Blume RS, MacLowry JD, Wolff SM: Limitations of chloride determination in the diagnosis of bromism. N Engl J Med 279:593, 1968
18. Murray T, Long W, Narins RG: Multiple myeloma and the anion gap. N Engl J Med 292:574, 1975
19. DeTroyer A, Stolarczyk A, DeBeyl DZ et al: Value of anion-gap determination in multiple myeloma. N Engl J Med 296:858, 1977
20. Winter SD, Pearson JR, Gabow PA et al: The fall of the serum anion gap. Arch Intern Med 150:311, 1990
21. Kulpmann WR: Influence of protein on the determination of sodium, potassium and chloride in serum by Ektachem DT 60 with the DTE module; evaluation with special attention to a possible protein error by flame atomic emission spectrometry and ion-selective electrodes; proposals to their calibration. J Clin Chem Clin Biochem 27:815, 1989
22. Panteghini M, Bonora R, Malchiodi A et al: Evaluation of the direct potentiometric method for serum chloride determination—comparison with the most commonly employed methodologies. Clin Biochem 19:20, 1986
23. Barlow IM, Harrison SP, Hogg GL: Evaluation of the Technicon Chem-1. Clin Chem 34:2340, 1988
24. Wrenn K: The delta (delta) gap: an approach to mixed acid-base disorders. Ann Emerg Med 19:1310, 1990
25. Mathias DW, Clifford PS, Klopfenstein HS: Mixed venous blood gases are superior to arterial blood gases in assessing acid-base status and oxygenation during acute cardiac tamponade in dogs. J Clin Invest 82:833, 1988
26. Widmer B, Gerhardt RE, Harrington JT et al: Serum electrolyte and acid-base composition. The influence of graded degrees of chronic renal failure. Arch Intern Med 139:1099, 1979
27. Kassirer JP, Schwartz WB: Correction of metabolic alkalosis in man without repair of potassium deficiency. Am J Med 40:19, 1966
28. Halperin ML, Hammeke M, Jose RG et al: Metabolic acidosis in the alcoholic: a pathophysiologic approach. Metabolism 32:308, 1983
29. Turino GM, Goldring RM, Heinemann HO: Renal response to mechanical ventilation in patients with chronic hypercapnia. Am J Med 56:151, 1974
30. Schwartz WB, Hays RM, Polak A et al: Effects of chronic hypercapnia on electrolyte and acid-base equilibrium. II. Recovery with special reference to the influence of chloride intake. J Clin Invest 40:1238, 1961
31. Pitts TO, Van Thiel DH: Disorders of the serum electrolytes, acid-base balance, and renal function in alcoholism. Recent Dev Alcohol 4:311, 1986
32. Alpern RJ, Stone DK, Rector FC Jr: Renal acidification mechanisms. p. 318. In Brenner BM, Rector FC Jr (eds): The Kidney. 4th Ed. WB Saunders, Philadelphia, 1991

8

Calcium Metabolism

Anthony Bleyer
Stanley Goldfarb

DISTRIBUTION

The body's calcium content is approximately 1 kg, with 6 g distributed in nonosseous tissues. Each day, the typical person consumes 900 mg of Ca (Fig. 8-1). Under the influence of 1,25 dihydroxy vitamin D (1,25 OH D), approximately 350 mg of Ca is absorbed in the gastrointestinal (GI) tract. One hundred and fifty milligrams is released with intestinal secretions, so that a net absorption of 200 mg is produced. The skeletal system takes up and releases approximately 200 to 400 mg of Ca each day in the course of remodelling. Therefore, approximately 200 mg of Ca must be excreted in the urine daily to maintain balance.

Calcium is distributed in the blood in either ionized (50%), protein-bound (40%), or complexed (10%) forms. Ionized Ca is the physiologically active component and is filtered by the glomerulus. Protein-bound Ca consists of Ca bound to albumin (0.8 mg Ca/g albumin) and globulin (0.18 mg Ca/g globulin). A decrease in albumin will result in a low total serum calcium, while the ionized calcium will remain normal. To correct for this discrepancy, one may use the following formula:

$$\text{Corrected serum Ca} = (4 - \text{serum albumin}) \times 0.8 + \text{serum Ca} \qquad \text{(Eq. 8-1)}$$

where 4 (g/dL) is the normal serum albumin. Alkalemia increases protein binding and lowers the total calcium, but ionized calcium is kept in the normal range through the actions of calcium-regulating hormones like PTH and Vitamin D. Complexed Ca consists of Ca bound to phosphate, bicarbonate, sulfate, and citrate. If the product of Ca and phosphate concentration (both in mg/dL) is greater than 60, calcium phosphate may precipitate in joints, vessels, skin, and the heart.

FUNCTION

Calcium has a structural and functional role. Structurally, 90% of the body's Ca is stored as hydroxyapatite in the bone. Calcium resorption and deposition is important in growth and the constant remodelling required to adapt to changing mechanical stresses.

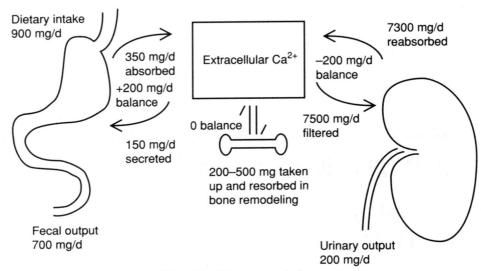

Fig. 8-1. Calcium metabolism.

Functionally, Ca is important in maintaining the electrical potential of each cell, modulating enzyme function, and serving as an important intracellular signalling mechanism.

REGULATION OF SERUM CALCIUM

Calcium metabolism is closely regulated by parathyroid hormone (PTH) and 1,25-dihydroxyvitamin D. In the absence of vitamin D and PTH, the plasma Ca is approximately 5.6 mg/dL (1.40 mEq/L); these hormones affect calcium balance such that the normal serum calcium is 10 mg/dL (2.5 mEq/L).

Parathyroid Hormone

Production

Parathyroid hormone is an 84–amino acid peptide important in the day-to-day maintenance of serum calcium (Fig. 8-2). It is produced and secreted by the parathyroid glands in response to hypocalcemia, and Ca exerts a negative feedback control on PTH.

Once produced, PTH is metabolized mainly in the liver to a 34 N terminal and a 50 C terminal peptide. The C peptide is inactive and slowly metabolized by the kidney through glomerular filtration. The N terminal peptide is the active moiety and is more rapidly metabolized by the kidney via mechanisms including glomerular filtration and peritubular uptake.

Actions

Parathyroid hormone acts predominantly on bone and kidney. Osteoblasts, but not osteoclasts, are known to have PTH receptors, and PTH stimulates osteoclast bone resorption through the indirect mediation of osteoblasts. Resorption of bone leads to transfer of Ca to the extracellular fluid (ECF), which results in a rising serum Ca.

The effect of PTH on the kidney is more complex (Fig. 8-3). Of the Ca filtered at the glomerulus, approximately 70% is reabsorbed in the proximal tubule in a manner closely linked to Na

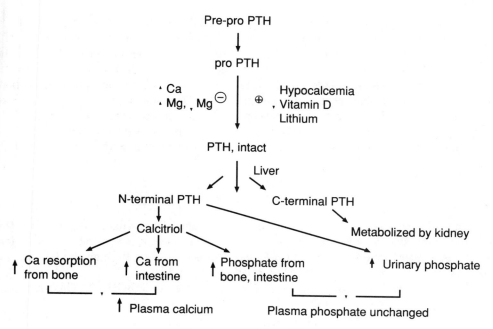

Fig. 8-2. PTH regulation.

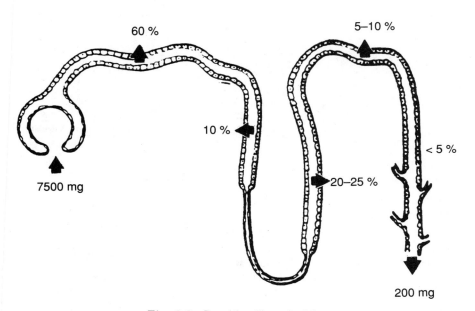

Fig. 8-3. Renal handling of calcium.

reabsorption and independent of PTH. Approximately 25% is reabsorbed in the pars recta and ascending limb of the loop of Henle. Here PTH has an effect at supraphysiologic doses. The remaining 10% to 15% is reabsorbed in the distal tubule under the influence of PTH. While promoting Ca reabsorption, PTH also has a phosphaturic effect, which is important because PTH action on bone releases phosphate and Ca. Without excretion of the phosphate, hyperphosphatemia could result, or phosphate could complex with Ca, resulting in a decrease in ionized Ca. Also, high serum phosphate actually antagonizes PTH action on bone.

PTH also has important effects on the proximal tubular cells, causing increased activity of 25-hydroxy vitamin D 1-alpha hydroxylase, which results in increased production of 1,25 OH D.

Vitamin D

FORMATION

In the skin, 7-dehydrocholesterol is converted by ultraviolet light to vitamin D_3, which is then transported to the kidney by vitamin D binding protein. The amount of sunlight needed to form vitamin D_3 is actually quite small. Vitamin D_3 may also be absorbed through the GI tract in a process that requires bile salts and micelle formation (Fig. 8-4).

In the liver, vitamin D_3 is converted to 25-hydroxy vitamin D (25 OH D). This step is not

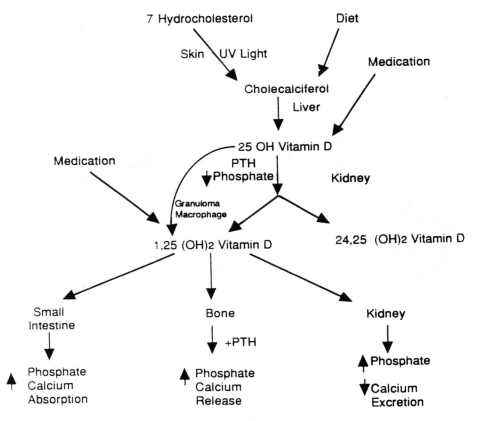

Fig. 8-4. Vitamin D regulation.

highly regulated. While 25 OH D has some of the functional characteristics of 1,25 OH D, it can only replace the latter when given in pharmacologic doses.

25 OH D may be metabolized to inactive forms by the cytochrome P450 system; any substances that increase the activity of this system decrease 25 OH D levels.

25 OH D is transported to the kidney via vitamin D binding protein or albumin. Here it undergoes conversion to 1,25 OH D. Conversion of 25 OH D to 1,25 OH D occurs in proximal tubule cells in a reaction mediated by 25-hydroxy vitamin D 1-alpha hydroxylase. Enzyme activity is enhanced by PTH and possibly hypophosphatemia, and decreased by increasing serum Ca, phosphate, and vitamin D levels.

Function

The vitamin D receptor has recently been characterized as a protein located in the nucleus, as would be expected for a steroid hormone. This protein has been found predominantly in the GI tract, the parathyroid gland, and in bone. In bone, receptors have been found on osteoblasts and not osteoclasts. Of note, receptors have also been found in the pancreas, testes, and ovaries, suggesting that many functions of vitamin D remain to be characterized. Also, many cancer cells have been found to express vitamin D receptors.

Vitamin D stimulates both Ca and phosphate absorption in the gut. When inserted into tissue culture, several hours are required for vitamin D–mediated transport to increase, which suggests that protein synthesis is required.

In the bone, vitamin D causes differentiation of the osteoclast cell line and Ca and phosphate resorption. Because of differing results from different cell lines, it is difficult to say if vitamin D has an anabolic effect on bone growth. However, it would appear that vitamin D is anabolic because its absence results in osteomalacia and rickets.

Vitamin D also binds to the parathyroid glands, and decreased 1,25 OH D, even in the presence of normocalcemia, will result in PTH production.

PTH and Vitamin D Interactions

It would seem that absence or overabundance of PTH or vitamin D would have little effect given the presence of the other hormone to counteract it. However, closer examination reveals a great interdependence between these two factors. First, PTH is needed for the production of 1,25 OH D. Second, an absence of vitamin D results in an obligatory overproduction of PTH, because of the vitamin D's effect on the parathyroid.

Other Hormones

Calcitonin is produced by the parafollicular cells of the parathyroid. Acute administration of calcitonin results in decreased activity of osteoclasts and decreased Ca resorption from bone. However, its role in chronic Ca homeostasis and bone metabolism appears minor, as patients who undergo thyroidectomy have no apparent abnormalities of bone composition or Ca homeostasis. 24, 25 OH D promotes bone mineralization and plays a minor role in GI absorption of calcium.

HYPERCALCEMIA

Symptoms

Hypercalcemia is frequently asymptomatic, and when symptoms are present, they are often nonspecific. As in most electrolyte disorders, the rate of change may be more important than the magnitude. The predominant effects of hypercalcemia involve the central nervous system, the kidney, and the neuromuscular system.

1. Confusion, lethargy, and obtundation frequently accompany hypercalcemia, especially in the aged. When hypercalcemia is chronic, patients may complain of anxiety, memory difficulties, and restlessness.
2. Loss of renal concentrating ability occurs, resulting first in polyuria and then volume depletion. These changes stimulate proximal Ca reabsorption and may worsen hypercalcemia. When associated with hyperparathyroidism or sarcoidosis, nephrolithiasis (kidney stones) may occur. This is to be distinguished from nephrocalcinosis, which is characterized by diffuse Ca deposits throughout the kidney. Nephrocalcinosis may occur with or without nephrolithiasis and is seen in chronic hypercalcemia, as well as medullary sponge kidney.

   Hypercalcemia also causes a reversible decrease in glomerular filtration rate (GFR), which may be due to tubular damage from Ca deposition or a direct vasoconstrictive action. This condition is characterized by a bland urinary sediment and absence of proteinuria. The decrease in GFR will reverse when hypercalcemia is corrected.
3. Constipation is common in hypercalcemic patients; anorexia, nausea, and vomiting may also occur.
4. Proximal muscle weakness may be quite marked. The finding of subacute progression of symmetrical proximal weakness is quite suggestive of hypercalcemia, particularly due to hyperparathyroidism.
5. Shortening of the QT interval may be present, and ventricular arrhythmias may occur with severe hypercalcemia.

Causes of Hypercalcemia

The most common cause of hypercalcemia is primary hyperparathyroidism, occurring in 250 patients per million each year. This condition may occur at any age but is classically encountered in older white females. Diagnosis rests on an elevated serum Ca and an elevated PTH. Eighty percent of cases are due to adenomas involving the gland, with the remainder predominantly resulting from hyperplasia. Hyperparathyroidism rarely is caused by parathyroid carcinoma.

Neoplasms are the second leading cause of hypercalcemia. The most common neoplasms causing hypercalcemia are carcinoma of the lung, breast cancer, multiple myeloma, lymphoma, and renal cell carcinoma. There are several mechanisms whereby tumors may cause hypercalcemia.

1. Direct invasion of the bone. Tumor cells may stimulate osteoclasts or directly produce Ca resorption.
2. Tumors may secrete a hormone known as PTH-related peptide. This substance's amino acid sequence is remarkably similar to PTH, and it has similar effects.
3. Tumors may release various substances that stimulate osteoclast resorption but have little effect on the kidney. These include transforming growth factor-α, lymphotoxin, tumor necrosis factor, and interleukin-1-α. Prostaglandins released from neoplasms may also cause bone resorption, though this is probably not clinically significant.

Vitamin D excess may result in hypercalcemia. Among the causes is overzealous vitamin D ingestion. Since vitamin D preparations are usually vitamin D_3 or 25 OH D, it is important to check 25 OH D levels in order to ascertain this diagnosis, as 1,25 OH D levels will be low or normal. Since 1,25 OH D is also available in tablet form, the 1,25 OH D level must also be checked.

Sarcoidosis and other granulomatous disorders can also link vitamin D and hypercalcemia.

Macrophages within granulomas produce 1,25 OH D alpha hydroxylase and stimulate production of 1,25 OH D. Other granulomatous disorders with similar mechanisms include tuberculosis, berrylliosis, histoplasmosis, and coccidiomycosis.

The milk alkali syndrome was prevalent when antacids and milk were used to treat peptic ulcer disease. Calcium is absorbed from milk and antacids, but, more importantly, the alkali from the antacids results in alkalemia, which reduces renal Ca excretion.

Endocrine disorders occasionally cause hypercalcemia. Thyrotoxicosis produces increased bone turnover, resulting in mild hypercalcemia. Pheochromocytomas and acromegaly may also cause hypercalcemia. Adrenal insufficiency may produce an increased serum Ca due primarily to increased protein binding of Ca and hemoconcentration; mild increases in ionized calcium may also occur. Multiple endocrine neoplasias (MEN) types I and II are associated with parathyroid neoplasia, which may result in hypercalcemia.

Immobilization may result in hypercalcemia, usually in association with other contributing factors, such as Paget's disease, renal insufficiency, or the rapid growth phase of adolescence.

Familial hypocalciuric hypercalcemia is an autosomal dominant condition in which patients have an increased serum Ca and almost always a normal PTH level. Hypophosphatemia and hypermagnesemia are also present. These patients are asymptomatic and do not respond to parathyroidectomy.

Some drugs also affect serum Ca levels. Lithium may cause mild increases in serum Ca by altering the set-point for PTH secretion. Thiazide diuretics may cause a 1 to 2 mg/dl increase in serum Ca. Once the thiazides are discontinued, Ca will return to normal over several weeks. Vitamin A in doses greater than 50,000 units/day will cause hypercalcemia, which may not resolve for several weeks after its discontinuation. Serum Ca can be normalized by giving glucocorticoids, as with vitamin D toxicity.

TREATMENT OF HYPERCALCEMIA

Intravenous saline is the essential element of hypercalcemia therapy. Most patients who present with hypercalcemia are volume depleted, resulting in marked proximal tubular reabsorption of Ca. Therefore, volume expansion is needed to inhibit proximal reabsorption and allow renal excretion of calcium. A dose of 4 to 5 L over 24 h, or more if this can be tolerated, is given. One must watch closely for signs of volume overload and congestive heart failure. The onset of action is immediate, and serum Ca will fall by 2 to 3 mEq/L over 8 to 24 hours. Relative contraindications to saline are renal failure and congestive heart failure.

Furosemide's diuretic effect allows for administration of increased amounts of saline and also blocks Ca reabsorption in the thick ascending limb. It can be used as an adjunct to saline, but used alone it is harmful because it causes volume contraction, thus increasing proximal reabsorption of Ca. The dosage is 40 to 80 mg po, or IV after volume status is corrected, titrated to effect. Volume depletion is a toxic side effect. The onset of action is immediate. Contraindications are renal failure and pre-existing volume depletion.

Calcitonin blocks osteoclast resorption and therefore decreases serum Ca. It is useful in the initial treatment of hypercalcemia, but tachyphylaxis develops within 2 to 3 days. Only salmon calcitonin has been approved for use in hypercalcemia. A test dose should be given to avoid potential allergic reactions. A standard dose is 4 British medical research council standard units per kilogram subcutaneously every 12 hours. Toxicity is allergic reactions, nausea, and flushing. The onset of action is from 2 to 4 hours. In 1 to 2 days, the decrease in serum Ca will be approximately 2 to 3 mg/dL. Allergy to calcitonin is a contraindication.

Mithramycin is an antineoplastic agent that was found to have a toxic effect on osteoclasts.

A dose of 25 μg/kg IV is given. Toxicity is nephrotoxicity, hepatotoxicity, nausea, and vomiting. Thrombocytopenia and increased prothrombin time may also occur. Nadir of serum calcium occurs in 1 to 2 days, and contraindications are renal insufficiency, thrombocytopenia, and hepatic failure.

Etidronate, and other biphosphonates such as pamidronate, are quickly becoming the agents of choice for hypercalcemia. These compounds, structurally similar to pyrophosphate, provide a significant decrease in serum calcium while also having few side effects. The dosage is 7.5 mg/kg/day given intravenously over several hours each day for 3 days. Toxicity is transient renal insufficiency, hyperphosphatemia, and renal failure with excessive or rapid dosing. The nadir is 4 to 7 days, and contraindication is renal insufficiency, with serum creatinine greater than 5 mg/dL.

Pamidronate (aminopropylidine diphosphonate) is a more potent diphosphonate and will most likely usurp etidronate in the management of hypercalcemia. The dosage is 60 or 90 mg intravenously over 24 h administered once. Toxicity is transient fever and leukopenia, usually during the first 2 days of treatment. Marked decrease in hearing was observed in two patients with otosclerosis. Nadir is 6 to 8 days, and a possible contraindication is otosclerosis.

Gallium nitrate is a recently approved agent that inhibits bone resorption, most likely through its effect on osteoclasts. The dosage is 200 mg/m^2, administered intravenously over 24 h for 5 days. Dosage may be terminated if hypercalcemia resolves. Toxicity is mild reversible renal insufficiency and hypophosphatemia. The nadir is 7 to 10 days, and contraindications are renal insufficiency and concurrent aminoglycoside administration.

Glucocorticoids are effective in decreasing serum Ca in hypercalcemic states resulting from hypervitaminosis A or D and sarcoidosis. They are also effective in hypercalcemia from hematologic malignancies.

Phosphates may be used to treat chronic hypercalcemia in hyperparathyroidism. They bind to Ca in the gut and prevent its absorption and bone resorption. Of note, oral phosphates cause diarrhea that frequently cannot be tolerated. Phosphates may cause systemic precipitation of calcium phosphate. They should not be given intravenously in hypercalcemic patients, and they should not be given orally if hyperphosphatemia is present.

Hemodialysis may be used to acutely lower serum Ca. It is most often indicated when acute renal failure is a complication of malignancy or hypercalcemia.

HYPOCALCEMIA

Clinical Manifestations

Neuromuscular irritability manifested by perioral numbness and carpopedal spasm is the hallmark of hypocalcemia. *Chvostek's sign* is produced by tapping on the cheek over the branches of the facial nerve. One observes the angle of the mouth for signs of muscle contraction. This sign is not specific, as it is frequently present in normal individuals. *Trousseau's sign* is produced by placing the blood pressure cuff over the forearm and raising the pressure to above the systolic pressure for 3 minutes. Carpal spasm will frequently be elicited when hypocalcemia is present.

Anxiety and depression may occur, as well as dementia in chronic conditions. Dry skin and coarse hair are other outward signs of hypocalcemia. A prolonged QT interval may be seen on the electrocardiogram, and basal ganglia calcification with extrapyramidal movement disorders may occur.

CAUSES OF HYPOCALCEMIA

Hypocalcemia is the epitomy of Murphy's Law: "Whatever can go wrong will go wrong." Any disorder that leads to decreased effective vitamin D or PTH can cause bone disease or hypocalcemia.

Disorders of PTH

Decreased PTH production, production of a nonfunctioning PTH, or deficient/defective PTH receptors may cause hypocalcemia. Decreased production of PTH can occur as a congenital, inherited, or acquired disorder.

1. DiGeorge's syndrome is caused by failure of development of the third and fourth branchial clefts. Absence of the thymus with attendant immunologic disorders and absence of the parathyroid glands occur. These patients present at birth with hypocalcemia.
2. Hypoparathyroidism may be inherited in a sex-linked, autosomal recessive, or autosomal dominant manner. It may present at any age.
3. Hypoparathyroidism may occur following thyroidectomy. For this reason, one must be vigilant in following symptoms and serum Ca postoperatively. Hypoparathyroidism has also occurred following radioactive iodine treatment for hyperthyroidism.
4. Idiopathic hypoparathyroidism can occur at any age. This disorder may be associated with alopecia, moniliasis, or Addison's disease.

An altered PTH peptide may be produced by the parathyroid gland, and, although being measured by assays, will not convey full functional effect. These patients will have normal PTH levels, but low urinary cAMP. They will respond to exogenous PTH.

There is a group of patients who produce a normal PTH but have end-organ resistance. This condition is known as pseudohypoparathyroidism type I. End-organ resistance may occur only at the bone or at the bone and kidney together. A subgroup of these patients characteristically are short in stature, have round faces, may suffer from mental retardation, and have brachydactyly of the fourth and fifth digits of the feet and hands. Patients who have this physical appearance and do not have end-organ resistance to PTH are said to have pseudopseudohypoparathyroidism.

Pseudohypoparathyroidism Type II patients show increased cAMP levels in response to their own PTH but still develop hypocalcemia and increased urinary calcium excretion.

Vitamin D Defects

Vitamin D_3 can be produced in the skin or absorbed in the GI tract. Both of these routes must be impaired in order to cause vitamin D deficiency. Markedly decreased exposure to the sun, especially in northern latitudes, will cause decreased vitamin D_3 synthesis. Lack of vitamin D in the diet is rare because of vitamin D supplementation in dairy products. However, malabsorption can result in vitamin D deficiency. Common conditions causing malabsorption include ileal bypass in the obese, short bowel syndrome, and blind loop syndromes. Of note, vitamin D undergoes significant enterohepatic recirculation, and if malabsorption is present, any parenteral vitamin D will also be lost in the stool.

Vitamin D_3 may not undergo 25 hydroxylation in the liver because of severe hepatic failure. More commonly, large doses of anticonvulsants such as phenytoin and phenobarbital increase the activity of the cytochrome P450 system, resulting in 25 OH D deficiency. Clinical vitamin D deficiency was frequently found in institutionalized individuals with seizure disorders.

Renal failure causes 1,25 OH D hydroxylase deficiency, resulting in normal 25 OH D levels, but very low 1,25 OH D. There is also an autosomal recessive 1,25 OH D enzyme deficiency, referred to as vitamin D–dependent rickets Type I. These patients will respond to 1,25 OH D administration.

In vitamin D–dependent rickets Type II, the vitamin D receptor is abnormal, and patients present with rickets despite normal or high 1,25 OH D levels.

Hypomagnesemia

Hypomagnesemia causes decreased response of the parathyroid gland to low serum Ca, decreased ability of the parathyroid gland to produce PTH, and decreased Ca exchange between bone and the extracellular fluid. Serum magnesium levels must be well below 1 mg/dl for this to occur.

Prostate Cancer

Metastatic prostate cancer markedly increases calcium deposition in the bone and may result in hypocalcemia.

CASE STUDY 1

Hypercalcemia Associated with Malignancy

A 64-year-old man is brought to the emergency room because of a 3-day history of progressive lethargy, obtundation, and weakness. Past medical history is unremarkable except for hypertension, for which the patient takes verapamil. The patient has a history of tobacco abuse. Physical examination reveals a disoriented afebrile patient with blood pressure 120/80 while lying flat and 90/50 while standing. The rest of the physical examination is notable for a heme negative stool with a prostate nodule on rectal examination. Neurologic examination reveals mild proximal muscle weakness.

LABORATORY DATA

Ca^{++} 15 mg/dL	Albumin 3.8 g/dL
PO_4 3.4 mg/dL	Creatinine 2.3 mg/dL
	BUN 78 mg/dL

Question 1. How do patients with hypercalcemia usually present?
Question 2. What symptoms are present in this case?
Question 3. What measures should be initiated?
Question 4. What diagnostic procedures should be initiated?

1. How do patients with hypercalcemia usually present?

In hypercalcemia of gradual onset (usually due to primary hyperparathyroidism), patients adjust to the slow increase in Ca and may have no or few symptoms. These patients may develop nephrolithiasis or simply complain of anorexia. They frequently have hypercalcemia detected on screening laboratory tests. This type of presentation is often seen with hyperparathyroidism or sarcoidosis. When the hypercalcemia is more acute, CNS symptoms are common, and patients are frequently lethargic or obtunded. This type of presentation is more common with neoplasms.

2. What symptoms are present in this case?

This patient has the common CNS manifestations of hypercalcemia, including lethargy and obtundation. Symmetrical proximal muscle weakness is also present, which is a clue to hypercalcemia and hyperparathyroidism.

Volume depletion is also common, due to decreased ability of the kidney to concentrate urine. There appear to be several factors involved, including an increase in prostaglandin production, which causes increased medullary flow. The increased blood flow can wash out the medullary gradient, resulting in decreased ability to conserve sodium and ultimately water. Volume contraction also increases proximal reabsorption of Ca, resulting in progressive hypercalcemia. Nausea and vomiting associated with the hypercalcemia also cause volume depletion, producing a vicious cycle.

The decrease in GFR seen in hypercalcemia is most likely due to Ca deposition in the tubules and interstitial inflammation but may also result from renal vasoconstriction. Decreased sensitivity to antidiuretic hormone is also present in hypercalcemia.

3. What measures should be initiated?

Volume expansion is of prime importance: 2 to 3 L of normal saline should be administered intravenously in the first 5 to 6 hours. Volume status should be followed closely, and if there is a history of cardiac disease, volume should be infused more slowly. Normal saline will decrease proximal reabsorption of calcium and enable more calcium to be excreted. After the patient's extracellular fluid volume is restored to normal, furosemide may be given. Furosemide decreases Ca reabsorption in the ascending limb of the loop of Henle and will increase urinary Ca excretion. It is important that furosemide is not given initially, as it may produce volume contraction, which is clearly deleterious.

In hypercalcemia associated with malignancy, humoral factors are frequently at work to decrease calcium excretion, limiting the benefit of volume expansion and furosemide. Therefore, it is important to also begin agents that will block osteoclastic resorption and thereby reduce bone release of calcium. Calcitonin is administered initially because it has the quickest onset of action and is the least toxic agent available. The most common side effects of calcitonin are nausea, vomiting, flushing, and allergic reactions.

First, a skin test of 10 international units (IU) is given on the forearm. Formation of a wheal or more than mild erythema is a contraindication to further treatment. If the skin test is negative, 4 IU/kg is then administered subcutaneously every 12 hours. This may be increased to 8 IU/kg every 6 hours. The majority of patients will respond within 2 hours of treatment. Therefore, after 5 to 6 hours, a repeat serum Ca should be obtained. If it appears there has been no response, vigorous treatment with saline and furosemide should continue, and the dosage may be increased. Tachyphylaxis to calcitonin occurs, and other agents are usually needed to control hypercalcemia chronically.

4. What diagnostic procedures should be initiated?

The most common causes of hypercalcemia are primary hyperparathyroidism and neoplasm, and these two conditions should be investigated first. Often the history will point to the other causes of hypercalcemia.

One may check for hyperparathyroidism by obtaining a PTH level. There are several determinations available, including N terminal, C terminal, and intact molecule assays. PTH is produced as an 84 amino acid peptide. The molecule is cleaved in the liver between amino acids 33 and 41 to produce an active N terminal component and an inactive C terminal peptide. The N terminal component is degraded rapidly by peritubular uptake and glomerular filtration. The C terminal peptides are inactive and accumulate in the blood; they are eventually degraded in the kidney by glomerular filtration. The C terminal assay recognizes the 30 carboxy-terminal amino acids. It will measure both the C terminal peptide and the intact molecule. Its value will be spurious in renal failure as the inactive C terminal metabolite is degraded more slowly when kidney function is decreased. The intact assay recognizes the tertiary structure of PTH as well as amino acids 28–48. It will therefore only recognize the intact molecule. The N terminal assay recognizes amino acids 1–34. It will measure the intact peptide as well as N terminal fragments. This patient with mild renal insufficiency should undergo measurement of PTH with either the intact or N terminal PTH assay. The results of this test will return in several days, so other possibilities of hypercalcemia are frequently ruled out in the interim.

When hypercalcemia is caused by malignancy, these neoplasms are usually quite obvious and will be detected on routine admission testing. The most common neoplasms causing hypercalcemia are squamous cell carcinoma of the lung, adenocarcinoma of the breast, squamous cell cancers of the head and neck, multiple myeloma, and renal cell carcinoma. Therefore, one may direct initial investigation toward these malignancies.

A history of bone pain will suggest myeloma, breast cancer, or lung cancer with bony metastases. On physical examination, a careful breast examination should be performed. Urinalysis should be checked for protein, and sulfosalicylic acid testing should be performed to detect light chains in the urine. A serum protein electrophoresis or a urine protein electrophoresis should be obtained to rule out myeloma.

A good posterior-anterior and lateral chest x-ray will investigate the possibility of lung cancer. Also, lymphadenopathy in the mediastinum will suggest T cell lymphoma or sarcoidosis. If resorption of the distal ends of the clavicles is seen, it suggests that the hypercalcemia is chronic in nature and may be due to hyperparathyroidism.

The patient's admitting chest x-ray revealed a large right hilar mass, centrally located. With volume repletion and calcitonin, serum Ca decreased to 12 mg/dL and serum creatinine decreased to 1 mg/dL.

Question 1. **What malignancies are associated with hypercalcemia, and is hypercalcemia a poor prognostic sign?**
Question 2. **What mechanisms are involved in the hypercalcemia of malignancy?**
Question 3. **What is the next step in the treatment of this patient's hypercalcemia?**

1. What malignancies are associated with hypercalcemia, and is hypercalcemia a poor prognostic sign?

Neoplasms frequently associated with hypercalcemia are squamous cell carcinoma of the lung, adenocarcinoma of the breast, multiple myeloma, prostate cancer, squamous cell carcinomas of the head and neck, renal cell carcinomas, ovarian cancer, and lymphoma. Rare cancers such as cholangiocarcinoma, VIPomas, and parathyroid carcinoma are frequently associated with hypercalcemia. Colon cancer and cervical cancer rarely cause hypercalcemia.

In general, patients with hypercalcemia from malignancy have a much poorer prognosis because disease is quite advanced at the time hypercalcemia occurs. In one study, 126 patients with hypercalcemia and various malignancies were examined. In patients with serum Ca measurements greater than 12 mg/dL, CNS symptoms occured in 80%, compared with 41% in patients with serum Ca levels below 12 mg/dL. If neoplasm-specific therapy could be administered, the median survival was 135 days, as compared with 30 days in patients who were not candidates for therapy. The median survival of patients with hematologic malignancies was 60 days. Treatment of hypercalcemia usually resulted in improvement in mental status.

Squamous cell carcinoma of the lung is associated with hypercalcemia in approximately 20% of cases. Small cell carcinoma is rarely associated with hypercalcemia. Almost all patients with hypercalcemia and squamous cell carcinoma are unresectable at the stage when hypercalcemia occurs. Metastases are frequently but not always present. The hypercalcemia is associated with markedly decreased survival, with median survival in one study of only one month.

Hypercalcemia associated with breast cancer is usually due to osteolytic metastases, and these patients also invariably have advanced disease and poor prognosis. Patients who have osteolytic metastases and do not have hypercalcemia have a much better survival than patients with metastases and hypercalcemia. In myeloma and renal cell carcinoma, hypercalcemia is also a poor prognostic sign.

2. What mechanisms are involved in the hypercalcemia of malignancy?

In general, there is decreased GI absorption of Ca, increased bone resorption, and increased renal reabsorption of Ca. PTH levels and vitamin D levels are usually, though not invariably, low. The findings differ from primary hyperparathyroidism because of decreased GI calcium absorption and decreased bone formation in general in hypercalcemia of malignancy.

Osteolytic metastases stimulate calcium resorption from bone through mechanisms that do not always involve osteoclasts. Tumor cells may recruit macrophages for this function or may reabsorb Ca from bone directly. Breast cancer typically causes hypercalcemia by bony metastases.

Several humoral factors have been identified to cause hypercalcemia. More than one of these may be present in each tumor. PTH-related peptide (PTHRP) is a protein whose genetic sequence is on chromosome 12 (PTH is produced on chromosome 11). The normal function of this protein is under investigation. PTHRP bears significant homology to PTH and stimulates osteoclasts, tubular reabsorption of calcium, and 1,25 OH D production. It is produced by squamous cell carcinoma of the head and neck, squamous cell carcinoma of the lung, and renal cell carcinoma.

Transforming growth factor-α is a potent stimulator of osteoclasts and produces hypercalcemia in many of the same tumors that produce PTHRP.

Lymphotoxin, tumor necrosis factor, interleukin-1-α and interleukin-1-β also stimulate bone resorption. Tumor prostaglandin production has been associated with hypercalcemia and bone resorption, though the importance of prostaglandins in hypercalcemia is controversial. In rare cases, prostaglandin inhibitors have appeared to decrease hypercalcemia, although these agents are usually unsuccessful.

Finally, some T cell and B cell lymphomas may have the capacity to produce 1,25 OH D from 25 OH D, resulting in hypercalcemia, though other mechanisms of hypercalcemia may also be involved in these disorders.

3. What is the next step in the treatment of this patient's hypercalcemia?

Calcitonin usually loses its efficacy over several days, and more potent agents are begun in anticipation. Etidronate is a biphosphonate that has a molecular structure similar to pyrophosphate. It binds to bone and prevents osteoclast resorption. Because of these properties, etidronate is being studied in Paget's disease, osteoporosis, and as a conservative therapy for hyperparathyroidism. It is also markedly effective in treating hypercalcemia. Etidronate may cause transient renal insufficiency, and it is contraindicated in patients with serum creatinine greater than 5 mg/dL. Tubular reabsorption of phosphate is increased with etidronate, and mild hyperphosphatemia may result. A dose of 7.5 mg/kg is infused intravenously over several hours each day for 3 consecutive days. Reduction in serum Ca occurs in 1 to 2 days, and a nadir is reached at 3 to 7 days. Approximately 50% of patients will become normocalcemic.

Another biphosphonate, pamidronate, has recently been introduced in the United States. In a double-blind, randomized trial in which patients received either pamidronate or etidronate, pamidronate normalized serum Ca levels in 70% of patients and etidronate in 41% ($P = .026$). Pamidronate is administered intravenously as a one-time dose of 60 or 90 mg via continuous infusion for 24 hours. Full response was usually achieved within 1 week, and duration of response was 1 to 31 days with a median value of 7 days. Side effects included fever, mild increases in serum creatinine, and phlebitis. Pamidronate therapy was associated with a subsequent fall in serum phosphate levels. A marked decrease in hearing acuity has occurred in two patients with otosclerosis who received pamidronate.

Gallium nitrate is another agent that has recently been introduced for the treatment of hypercalcemia, decreasing bone resorption through an osteoclast-mediated mechanism. Mild, reversible increases in serum creatinine have been reported, and gallium nitrate is therefore contraindicated in patients with renal insufficiency or in patients receiving aminoglycosides. Patients receive 200 mg/m^2 over 24 hours for up to 5 days. Dosage is terminated when normocalcemia appears. Onset of action and duration of response is similar to the biphosphonates.

Mithramycin may also be used as treatment for hypercalcemia, though its toxicity is greater than that of etidronate. It was initially developed as a chemotherapeutic agent, effective in the treatment of testicular cancer. During initial studies, mithramycin was found to lower serum Ca, and it has since been studied for this indication. Its action appears to be that of decreasing osteoclast activity, probably by DNA intercalation with subsequent cell death. Patients receiving mithramycin may develop nausea and vomiting. Hepatotoxicity and nephrotoxicity may also occur. Therefore, the drug is contraindicated in hepatic failure and renal insufficiency. Thrombocytopenia and an increase in fibrinolytic activity, associated with an increased prothrombin time, may also occur. These toxicities are more common when the drug is used at higher doses to treat malignancies. The recommended dosage for hypercalcemia is 25 μg/kg, which may be repeated if there is no improvement in serum Ca in 24 to 48 hours. The improvement in serum Ca may last up to 2 weeks. Mithramycin is probably somewhat less effective than etidronate.

Definitive therapy of hypercalcemia requires treatment of the underlying malignancy. It is essential that these patients remain volume-repleted to avoid further increases in serum Ca.

CASE STUDY 2

Hypercalcemia Associated with Hyperparathyroidism

A 58-year-old woman presents to your office after routine screening laboratory tests revealed a serum Ca of 12 mg/dL. She is asymptomatic and wants to know "what the big deal is," as she feels well.

Question 1. Is primary hyperparathyroidism a likely cause, and why is family history important in this regard?

Question 2. What other conditions are associated with hypercalcemia, and what questions should be emphasized in the history?

Question 3. What laboratory tests should be ordered in the ambulatory, hypercalcemic patient?

Question 4. Are other tests needed for the diagnosis of primary hyperparathyroidism?

Question 5. How is a parathyroidectomy performed?

Question 6. What alternatives are there for ablation of parathyroid tissue?

Question 7. Does every patient with primary hyperparathyroidism require parathyroidectomy?

Question 8. If conservative medical treatment is employed, what should be monitored, and what medications may be of benefit?

---

1. **Is primary hyperparathyroidism a likely cause, and why is family history important in this regard?**

The most common cause of hypercalcemia in the ambulatory setting is primary hyperparathyroidism. This condition occurs twice as frequently in women as in men, and is most common after menopause. The patient may have a history of renal calculi, or have any of the presenting symptoms of hypercalcemia. Due to frequent laboratory testing in the general population, hyperparathyroid patients are usually diagnosed when they are asymptomatic. In some cases, patients will present with nephrolithiasis. Primary hyperparathyroidism is quite common, with a prevalence of 1 in 1000.

Primary hyperparathyroidism is caused by a parathyroid adenoma in approximately 80% of cases. In 20% the cause will be parathyroid hyperplasia involving all four glands. Parathyroid carcinoma is a rare condition that may also cause hypercalcemia. The increased PTH production that results from these conditions causes increased renal Ca reabsorption and increased resorption of Ca from bone. Increased excretion of phosphate in the urine is also present. PTH and hypophosphatemia also stimulate 1,25 OH D production, resulting in increased gastrointestinal absorption of Ca. The increase in bone resorption usually causes increased Ca delivery to the kidney, overwhelming the PTH-induced Ca reabsorption, with the result of hypercalciuria. In primary hyperparathyroidism there is usually some feedback control and serum Ca remains relatively stable on a day-to-day basis. Over time, the hyperparathyroidism may worsen and serum Ca may slowly rise. Rarely, there will be a dramatic increase in serum Ca resulting in increased symptomatology. Patients may develop nephrolithiasis from the increased excretion of Ca and phosphate. Also, continued bone resorption may result in osteitis fibrosa et cystica—a skeletal condition characterized by subperiosteal bone resorption and bone demineralization, as well as the occurrence of bony cysts. This condition is dramatically exemplified by the case of Charles Martell, a large, healthy seaman, who was 6'1" before he developed hyperparathyroidism. Over the course of several years he lost 7 inches in height, sustained multiple fractures, and suffered from nephrolithiasis. He was the first patient with hyperparathyroidism who was presented in the literature, in work performed by Dr. Fuller Albright at the Massachusetts General Hospital in the 1920s.

Patients with hyperparathyroidism may develop any of the symptoms of hypercalcemia, including bone pain, fatigue, and anorexia. There may be an increased incidence of peptic ulcer disease and hypertension in these patients. Again, it must be emphasized that many patients are asymptomatic and with follow-up frequently remain without complaint.

Diagnosis relies on an elevated PTH level in the presence of hypercalcemia. PTH stimulates production of cyclic AMP in the urine, and one may measure urinary cAMP, though this is less specific. Hypophosphatemia is seen in 50% of these patients. PTH may stimulate bicarbonate wasting, and patients with hyperparathyroidism usually have a serum chloride of greater than 100 mEq/L, while hypercalcemia from other causes is usually associated with a serum chloride less than 100 mEq/L. The usefulness of this test is limited, as there is definite overlap between these conditions. Patients with hyperparathyroidism frequently have hypercalciuria because the bone resorption of Ca overwhelms the increased renal tubular reabsorption of Ca.

One should inquire specifically about a family history of hyperparathyroidism or hypercalcemia, as 10% of cases will be familial. Multiple endocrine neoplasia Type I (MEN 1) is an autosomal dominant condition that is almost always associated with parathyroid hyperplasia. Other manifestations include tumors of the pituitary and pancreatic islet cells. MEN 2, also an autosomal dominant condition, consists of pheochromocytomas, medullary carcinoma of the thyroid, and parathyroid hyperplasia. Parathyroid involvement is not as common as in MEN 1.

A family history of hypercalcemia without hyperparathyroidism suggests familial hypercalcemic hypocalciuria. These patients have mild elevations of serum Ca and are almost always asymptomatic and without nephrolithiasis. Occasionally, patients have pancreatitis, which may be related to the hypercalcemia. The cause of this autosomal dominant condition is under investigation. There may be increased sensitivity of the kidney to PTH, or increased absorption of Ca in the ascending limb of the loop of Henle. Patients usually have serum Ca measurements in the same range as patients with primary hyperparathyroidism (10–14 mg/dL). The clue to this condition is a low daily urinary calcium excretion, usually 80–100 mg/24 h. Serum PTH levels are normal, but may occasionally be mildly elevated. If these patients undergo parathyroidectomy, their serum Ca will not change, unless the surgery involves removal of all parathyroid glands. As this condition almost never has any adverse manifestations, these patients should be spared a partial parathyroidectomy, which will be ineffective, or a total parathyroidectomy, which will produce hypoparathyroidism.

In some cases it may not be possible to distinguish familial hypercalcemic hypocalciuria from early primary hyperparathyroidism. Both conditions may be associated with hypercalcemia, low 24-hour urinary calcium measurements, and mildly elevated PTH. In this instance, both parents and siblings should be tested. If family members cannot be tested, one may follow the patient. Primary hyperparathyroidism may worsen, but familial hypercalcemic hypocalciuria will not. Also, the latter condition is present since birth, so that previous normal serum Ca levels tend to negate this diagnosis.

2. What other conditions are associated with hypercalcemia, and what questions should be emphasized in the history?

Medications often cause hypercalcemia, and one should carefully question patients in this regard. Thiazide diuretics increase distal nephron reabsorption of calcium and bone resorption, and patients may occasionally develop mild hypercalcemia. If this occurs, the medication should be discontinued, and serum Ca rechecked in 2 to 3 weeks. One should be careful to exclude other contributing factors such as early primary hyperparathyroidism. Lithium may cause a mild increase in PTH production due to an altered set-point for PTH release. Again, the serum Ca is usually only mildly elevated.

The physician needs to ask directly about vitamin usage, as many patients will not consider vitamins medications and may be embarassed by their excessive vitamin intake. Vitamin D toxicity is usually caused by increased exogenous vitamin D_2, the common form of vitamin D used in supplements. However 25 OH D and 1,25 OH D are also available, and one must consider them as a potential source of toxicity. The normal daily requirement is 100 to 200 IU per day. When patients receive greater than 50,000 IU per day, toxicity may occur. The only foods with naturally concentrated vitamin D_3 are the livers of certain fish, so that one may become vitamin D intoxicated only by ingestion of vitamins. Vitamin D_3 is hydroxylated in the liver to 25 OH D in a reaction that is not closely regulated. 25 OH D then undergoes 1-hydroxylation in the kidney in a closely regulated reaction. Therefore, exogenous vitamin D intake will result in high 25 OH D levels but normal or low 1,25 OH D levels. The appropriate test to ascertain this diagnosis is therefore a 25 OH D level. A 1,25 OH D level should also be obtained, as 1,25 OH D is also available as an oral medication. Patients may develop all the complications of hypercalcemia and may develop irreversible renal toxicity leading to renal failure. Once the diagnosis is made, the vitamins should be stopped. The half-life of 25 OH D is quite long, so that hypercalcemia may not improve for several weeks. Also, patients sometimes may continue to ingest vitamin D, despite claims to the contrary. One may give prednisone, 40 to 60 mg per day, which will correct the hypercalcemia prior to a decrease in 25 OH D levels. Prednisone may actually be used as a diagnostic trial in any cases of hypercalcemia believed due to increased vitamin D.

Other conditions associated with increased vitamin D are granulomatous conditions such as sarcoidosis, berylliosis, tuberculosis, and coccidiomycosis. Macrophages in these granulomas possess the ability to hydroxylate 25 OH D. Again prednisone may be used diagnostically and therapeutically, though it should be avoided in tuberculosis.

Vitamin A toxicity also causes hypercalcemia when ingested in doses greater than 50,000 units per day. To make the diagnosis one should measure vitamin A levels. This condition also responds to treatment with prednisone.

Another medication that may be forgotten unless specifically addressed is antacids. Milk and antacids were commonly used to treat peptic ulcer disease. Milk contains Ca and vitamin D, but more importantly, antacids contain alkali, which can cause a mild metabolic alkalosis. Bicarbonate increases Ca reabsorption in the distal tubule, and therefore patients ingesting large amounts of these agents can develop hypercalcemia.

Thyrotoxicosis may also result in hypercalcemia so one should inquire about heat intolerance, weight loss, and decreased need for sleep. Thyrotoxicosis causes increased bone turnover, which leads to the hypercalcemia. Other endocrine disorders that may rarely cause mild hypercalcemia include pheochromocytoma and acromegaly. Addison's disease causes an increase in total serum Ca due to increased protein binding. Mild increases in ionized Ca are occasionally seen.

Immobilization may result in hypercalcemia, usually in adolescents in their rapid growth phase or patients with renal insufficiency or Paget's disease.

Patients with hypercalcemia associated with advanced chronic liver disease have been reported. These patients had a mean total bilirubin concentration of 29.5 mg/dL. In most of the patients, PTH, 25 OH D, and 1,25 OH D were normal or in the low normal range.

3. What laboratory tests should be ordered in the ambulatory, hypercalcemic patient?

On the initial visit, a serum Ca and phosphorus should be repeated. A serum creatinine should be obtained to check for renal insufficiency. An N terminal PTH, C terminal PTH, or intact PTH assay should be ordered, and a 25 OH D level or a 1,25 OH D level may be obtained if there is a suspicion of exogenous vitamin D or granulomatous disease respectively.

In our patient, the serum PTH returns markedly elevated and the serum Ca is 13 mg/dL, serum phosphate 3.0 mg/dL, and serum creatinine 1.0 mg/dL.

4. Are other tests needed for the diagnosis of primary hyperparathyroidism?

The above laboratory tests assure us that primary hyperparathyroidism is present. One may obtain an abdominal x-ray to rule out nephrolithiasis, as this may affect further management.

The patient states she has heard that she will need a parathyroidectomy and wants to know the morbidity of this procedure.

5. How is a parathyroidectomy performed?

The procedure involves exploration of the four glands to find the single adenoma causing hyperparathyroidism in 80% of affected patients. Twenty percent of the cases will be due to hyperplasia of the four glands, and a small percentage (about 3%) will have more than one adenoma. If the surgeon localizes the adenoma on the first side explored, the wound is closed and the other side is not examined. If diffuse hyperplasia is present, three and one-half of the glands are usually removed. The remaining glandular tissue may be transplanted to the forearm for easier access in case further tissue removal is required. Often, some tissue is cryopreserved in case of a complication with transplantation.

Parathyroid tissue is not always easily localized to the thyroid. If an adenoma cannot be found, and all four glands cannot be identified, exploration of the retropharyngeal or retroesophageal spaces is undertaken. The thymus is removed, as this will contain the parathyroid in 10% of the cases. If normal glands are found on one side, and the adenoma cannot be found, the contralateral half of the thyroid is removed, as the parathyroid glands may be deeply embedded.

If there is no success in finding the adenoma, the wound is closed, and localization is performed. The wound may be re-opened in about 7 weeks.

Localization is usually done after a failed parathyroidectomy but may be done before the first exploration to minimize duration of anesthesia if the patient is a surgical risk. Also, localization may be attempted if the hypercalcemia is severe, and it is felt that the patient cannot tolerate hypercalcemia for 6 weeks in the event the initial parathyroidectomy attempt is unsuccessful.

Localization may be performed with high-resolution CT scanning, ultrasound, thallium-technetium scanning, MRI, or angiography. The efficacy of these techniques varies. CT scanning appears to be quite successful, but angiography with highly selective venous catheterization is the most accurate modality. The success of parathyroidectomy is closely related to the experience and skill of the surgeon.

6. What alternatives are there for ablation of parathyroid tissue?

Percutaneous injection of parathyroid adenomas with alcohol after localization with ultrasound is being investigated as an alternative approach to parathyroidectomy. Possible complications would include danger to the recurrent laryngeal nerve, which is situated near the parathyroid glands. Localization of the gland with angiography and installation of full-strength contrast into the gland through an adjacent artery has been tried, but this procedure has been complicated by acute cerebrovascular accidents.

7. Does every patient with primary hyperparathyroidism require parathyroidectomy?

This question is most difficult to answer. There are several potential hazards of hyperparathyroidism. First, bone resorption occurs, and it is feared patients are more likely to develop osteoporosis. Also, hyperparathyroidism has been associated with increased cardiovascular mortality and possibly increased mortality from cancer. Patients may develop worsening hypercalcemia or nephrolithiasis and require the procedure at a later date if not done initially. Also, the surgical risk of parathyroidectomy is quite low. Patients treated conservatively will require long-term follow-up; after 6 years the cost of tests and follow-up will equal that of parathyroidectomy. On the other hand, the incidence of primary hyperparathyroidism has increased simply due to abnormal laboratory findings in asymptomatic patients. Whether surgical intervention will change the life of these asymptomatic patients has not been determined. Several centers are now following asymptomatic patients to determine if conservative therapy is adequate. There has been difficulty obtaining careful follow-up in these patients, but many appear to remain asymptomatic without significant change in bone density and without the development of nephrolithiasis.

8. If conservative medical treatment is employed, what should be monitored, and what medications may be of benefit?

The patient should have initial bone densitometry and abdominal x-ray (to check for nephrolithiasis or nephrocalcinosis). Follow-up should occur every 6 to 12 months, with careful monitoring for symptoms, repeating serum Ca, phosphate, and PTH measurements, and bone density serially evaluated by dual photon absorptiometry.

Estrogens and progestins may be helpful in conservative therapy. These hormones decrease calcium resorption from bone and may inhibit osteoporosis. Serum Ca and urinary Ca excretion also decrease.

Oral phosphates will decrease GI absorption of Ca and will raise serum phosphate levels. Since 1,25 OH D production is stimulated by hypophosphatemia, 1,25 OH D levels will fall. However, PTH and urinary cAMP levels increase, and these changes may offset any benefit of decreased vitamin D levels. This treatment remains under investigation.

CASE STUDY 3

Symptoms of Hypocalcemia

A 21-year-old woman presents to the emergency room complaining of numbness and tingling in her hands and feet. She states she has been quarreling with her boyfriend and appears quite hysterical. Her pulse is 100 beats per minute, regular. Her blood pressure is 100/70 mmHg, and her respiratory rate is 34 per minute. She is complaining of muscle spasms in her feet.

Question 1. Are this patient's symptoms consistent with hypocalcemia?
Question 2. What may be contributing to a disturbance in serum Ca in this patient?
Question 3. How can this diagnosis be made definitively?

1. Are this patient's symptoms consistent with hypocalcemia?

The hallmark of hypocalcemia is tetany, which is characterized by peri-oral numbness, tingling of the hands and feet, and carpopedal spasm. Patients may even develop seizures. Anxiety and depression may occur, and dementia may be present in chronic hypocalcemia. Tetany may be induced by several maneuvers. The physician should inflate the blood pressure cuff over the forearm to just over systolic pressure for three minutes. If hypocalcemia is present, the hand will spasm. A positive result is referred to as Trousseau's sign. Also, the physician should attempt to elicit Chvostek's sign, which involves tapping on the facial nerve to elicit muscle contraction. One should lightly percuss approximately 1 cm below the zygomatic process of the temporal bone, 2 cm anterior to the ear lobe. This direct mechanical stimulation will result in contraction of the facial muscles and will be enhanced by hypocalcemia. A mild response will consist of twitching at the angle of the mouth. This response will be present in up to 25% of normocalcemic individuals, so its presence is very nonspecific. A stronger response occurs when the mouth and alar nasae both contract, though this response, too, may occasionally still be seen in normal individuals. If contraction of the orbicularis oculi or the forehead musculature occurs, the diagnosis of hypocalcemia is quite certain. Trousseau's sign has more clinical utility than Chvostek's sign, though neither sign may be present in some patients with hypocalcemia. Chronic hypocalcemia may also cause basal ganglial calcifications, and patients may display extra-pyramidal movement disorders.

Other features of hypocalcemia include dry skin and coarse hair. Cardiac conduction abnormalities may also occur, and the electrocardiogram may reveal a prolonged QT interval.

The anxiety, perioral numbness, tingling of extremities and muscle spasm in this patient are consistent with hypocalcemia.

2. What may be contributing to a disturbance in serum Ca in this patient?

Calcium is distributed within the blood as protein-bound (40%), complexed (10%), and ionized Ca (50%). Calcium binds predominantly with albumin (0.8 mg Ca/g albumin), with lesser binding to globulins (0.18 mg Ca/g globulin). In the blood, Ca also complexes with phosphate, sulfate, and citrate. The ionized Ca is the metabolically active component, and changes in protein binding may result in decreases in ionized Ca.

In this patient, hyperventilation has likely induced a respiratory alkalosis. The rise in systemic pH per se is primarily responsible for her neurologic symptoms. The rise in blood pH induced by respiratory alkalosis also increases Ca binding to albumin and phosphate, and acutely reduces the ionized Ca, further contributing to the neurologic symptoms.

3. How can this diagnosis be made definitively?

If the total serum Ca is measured, results may be low in the presence of a normal ionized Ca. This usually occurs because the serum albumin is low. One may correct the serum Ca by subtracting the patient's albumin from 4 (the normal serum albumin) and multiplying the result by 0.8. This number is then added to the patient's Ca to result in the corrected serum Ca.

$$\text{Corrected serum Ca}^{++} = (4\text{-serum albumin}) \times 0.8 + \text{serum Ca}^{++} \qquad \text{(Eq. 8-2)}$$

However, in this patient, this still will not help us to determine the ionized Ca, as the above formula does not take into account changes in protein binding due to changes in pH. Therefore, one could order a serum ionized Ca. This measurement is performed with a Ca-selective electrode; the result can frequently be obtained before the serum Ca is performed. However, it is more cost-effective to await a recovery of her emotional composure to determine if the symptoms persist beyond that point. If they do, the ionized Ca can be measured.

The patient's ionized Ca returns at 0.95 mEq/L (normal 1.00–1.25 mEq/L). The patient is reassured and comforted. Her respiratory rate returns to normal, and her symptoms resolve.

CASE STUDY 4

Hypocalcemia Associated with Alcoholism

An elderly patient presents to the emergency room with complaints of fever, tremulousness, and diarrhea. The patient's history is remarkable for alcoholism and a seizure disorder. Physical examination is significant for a temperature of 39.5°C, abdominal tenderness, and the presence of Chvostek's and Trousseau's signs. Urinalysis reveals many gram negative rods and pyuria. An ionized Ca is measured and returns at 0.85 mEq/L (normal 1.00–1.25 mEq/L). The patient is admitted to the intensive care unit, and you are called as a consultant to explain the significance of a low serum ionized Ca.

Question 1.   How is the ionized Ca interpreted?
Question 2.   What are the most common causes of hypocalcemia in critically ill patients and what are likely causes of hypocalcemia in this patient?
Question 3.   What are the other causes of hypocalcemia?

---

1. How is the ionized Ca interpreted?

Most clinicians are familiar with the serum Ca (measured in mg/dL) and feel they do not have a "clinical sense" for the value of an ionized Ca. Part of the problem is that serum Ca is usually measured in mg/dl, and ionized Ca is measured in mEq/L. The normal total serum Ca is 8.5 to 10.5 mg/dL, which corresponds to 2.13 to 2.62 mEq/L. Since ionized Ca is approximately 50% of serum Ca, a normal ionized Ca will usually be approximately 1.06 to 1.31 mEq/L.

2. What are the most common causes of hypocalcemia in critically ill patients, and what are likely causes of hypocalcemia in this patient?

Hypocalcemia may be present in as many as 70% of patients admitted to medical intensive care units. The most common causes of hypocalcemia in this setting are renal insufficiency, hypomagnesemia, and sepsis.

Renal failure results in decreased production of 1,25 OH D, and increased serum concentrations of phosphate. These two factors frequently cause hypocalcemia in patients with end-stage renal disease who are noncompliant or not receiving adequate follow-up.

Hypomagnesemia results from a decreased response of the parathyroid gland to hypocalcemia, decreased ability of the parathyroid gland to produce PTH, and decreased Ca exchange within the bone. Common causes of hypomagnesemia include loop diuretics, chronic diarrhea and inflammatory bowel disease, and antibiotics such as aminoglycosides and amphotericin B. Alcoholics frequently suffer from hypomagnesemia because of increased renal excretion of Mg due to ethanol, diets poor in Mg, and vomiting and diarrhea. Serum Mg values less than 1 mg/dL may be responsible for hypocalcemia. Another manifestation of hypomagnesemia is hypokalemia. Hypermagnesemia also causes hypocalcemia by decreasing the threshold for PTH secretion.

Sepsis, usually in association with gram-negative organisms or toxic shock syndrome, may result in hypocalcemia. The mortality of patients with hypocalcemia and sepsis is higher than in patients with sepsis alone. Sepsis appears to cause decreased production of PTH, decreased production of 1,25 OH D by the kidney, and resistance to the actions of 1,25 OH D. Endotoxin may mediate some of these changes. In toxic shock syndrome, markedly elevated calcitonin levels may be present.

Medications such as phenytoin and phenobarbital increase the activity of the cytochrome P450 system in the liver. This may result in metabolism of 25 OH D and resultant hypocalcemia.

Given this patient's history, sepsis, hypomagnesemia from alcohol intake and diarrhea, and anticonvulsant therapy may be causes of hypocalcemia.

3. What are the other causes of hypocalcemia?

The list of conditions causing hypocalcemia is rather lengthy. The easiest way to remember them is to go through PTH and vitamin D formation and action, and consider where these pathways may be interrupted.

PTH is formed in the parathyroid gland and then exerts its actions primarily at the bone and kidney. Deficiencies of PTH production are caused by a nonfunctioning parathyroid gland and may be congenital, inherited, or idiopathic.

Congenital absence of the parathyroid gland will result in neonatal hypocalcemia. DiGeorge syndrome causes a failure of development of the third and fourth branchial clefts. Patients suffer from absence of the parathyroid gland as well as absence of the thymus, resulting in severe immunologic disorders and hypocalcemia.

Hypoparathyroidism may be inherited as an autosomal dominant, autosomal recessive, or sex-linked condition and may present at any age.

Idiopathic hypoparathyroidism occurs as an isolated condition or may be associated with moniliasis, Addison's disease, alopecia, diabetes, or pernicious anemia. The condition presents in childhood and appears to be autoimmune in nature.

Hypoparathyroidism may also result from invasion of the glands by tumors, amyloidosis, or sarcoidosis. Parathyroid glands may be injured by radioactive iodine therapy for thyrotoxicosis. Following thyroidectomy, the patient must be followed closely for loss of parathyroid glands. The Chvostek sign should be checked preoperatively, and if not present may be used to follow the patient postoperatively.

Some patients will produce an amount of PTH measurable by immunoassays, but still nonfunctional because of changes in the amino acid sequence. These patients will have normal PTH levels, but hypocalcemia and low urinary cAMP levels. Their urinary cAMP will increase when they are administered exogenous PTH, and Ca metabolism will return to normal.

If PTH production is intact, one should consider resistance of bone and kidney to the effects of PTH. Pseudohypoparathyroidism Type I is associated with normal PTH production, but lack of PTH function. These patients will suffer from hypocalcemia and have normal PTH levels.

However, they will not respond to exogenous PTH. Lack of receptor function may occur only at the bone or at the bone and kidney. A subgroup of these patients will be of short stature, have round faces, suffer from mental retardation, and have brachydactyly of the fourth and fifth digits of the hands and feet. Patients who have these physical features but do not have hypocalcemia are said to have pseudopseudohypoparathyroidism.

Pseudohypoparathyroidism Type II patients have normal urinary cAMP levels but still have hypocalcemia and increased urinary calcium excretion. They will not respond to exogenous PTH.

Defects of vitamin D must then be considered. Vitamin D is a lipid-soluble vitamin that may be absorbed through the GI tract or made in the skin in the presence of ultraviolet radiation. Both systems must fail for vitamin D deficiency to occur. The only naturally occurring fortified source of vitamin D is the liver of certain fish. However, in the United States milk and dairy products are fortified with vitamin D, making dietary deficiency extremely uncommon. Problems with vitamin D deficiency occur because of malabsorption, which occurs in blind loop syndrome, short bowel syndrome, and ileal bypass for obesity. If there is no GI absorption of vitamin D, sunlight is needed for production of vitamin D. The amount of sunlight required is minimal, but more sunlight is needed in northern climates and with dark-skinned individuals.

Vitamin D_3 is present in the diet and produced in the skin in the presence of sunlight. This molecule must then undergo 25 hydroxylation in the liver. In cases of severe hepatic failure, 25 hydroxylation may not occur. More common, however, is increased metabolism of 25 OH D when the cytochrome P450 system's activity is increased by phenytoin or phenobarbital.

The next step in formation is the 1 hydroxylation that occurs in the kidney. This step will not occur in the presence of renal failure. Also, there is an autosomal recessive form of 1 hydroxylase deficiency. These patients have vitamin D–dependent rickets Type 1, and their rickets can be corrected by administration of 1,25 OH D. Patients suffer from bone pain, skeletal deformities including genu varus, and myopathy.

Patients with vitamin D–dependent rickets Type 2 have normal levels of 1,25 OH D, but their vitamin D receptors do not function correctly.

There are several other causes of hypocalcemia. Pancreatitis causes calcium deposition in the kidney and possibly inactivation of PTH. Rhabdomyolysis results in phosphate leakage from damaged muscle cells, causing calcium phosphate deposition and hypocalcemia. The acquired immunodeficiency syndrome has been associated with hypocalcemia, although the mechanism is unclear. Patients with AIDS who are treated with foscarnet (trisodium phosphonoformate) for cytomegalovirus retinitis may develop hypocalcemia due to chelation of foscarnet with calcium.

Massive red blood cell transfusions may cause hypocalcemia. First, the tremendous volume expansion with Ca-poor fluid provokes hypocalcemia. Second, the red blood cells contain citrate as a preservative. When the blood is transfused, the citrate leaks into the extracellular fluid and complexes with Ca.

Osteoblastic metastases in prostate cancer may stimulate marked Ca deposition and cause hypocalcemia in this manner.

Finally, patients with renal failure who undergo parathyroidectomy may develop marked hypocalcemia. Typically, these patients have had elevated PTH levels for several years, resulting in chronic depletion of Ca from the bones. After parathyroidectomy, for the first time there is an unopposed ability to deposit Ca in bones that are markedly depleted. This "hungry bone syndrome" may last several weeks and requires intensive monitoring of serum Ca and frequent infusions of Ca.

Further history reveals that the patient has recently continued marked alcohol consumption. Blood cultures return positive for *Escherichia coli,* and a diagnosis of urosepsis is confirmed. The serum Mg level returns at 0.4 mg/dL. Magnesium stores are repleted, antibiotic therapy is begun, and several days later the serum Ca has returned to normal.

CASE STUDY 5

Hypocalcemia Post-Parathyroidectomy

As the nephrology consultant you are called to see a patient who underwent parathyroidectomy 3 days ago and is now having seizures. His serum Ca has been measured and is 5 mg/dL with a normal serum albumin. An obviously distraught and anxious house officer asks you what to do.

Question 1. What treatment should be initiated?

---

1. What treatment should be initiated?

Seizures associated with hypocalcemia may take one of two forms. They may appear as severe tetany followed by several clonic contractions. Patients may remain conscious during these episodes and will not lose control of their bladder. Patients will also suffer typical generalized seizures—as well as petit-mal and focal seizures—in association with hypocalcemia. Phenytoin has been effective in both types of seizures and should not be withheld simply because of hypocalcemia.

Correction of the hypocalcemia should always be done intravenously if the cause of hypocalcemia is not known, as vitamin D levels may be low, and absorption of calcium from the GI tract will not occur. If vitamin D levels are low, one may actually give oral Ca in doses of greater than 4 g a day, and Ca will be absorbed by diffusion. One may administer either calcium chloride or calcium gluconate parenterally. Calcium chloride may cause venous sclerosis and should only be administered centrally; calcium gluconate is, therefore, usually preferable. One should anticipate administering approximately 300 mg of Ca to control tetany. Over 5 to 10 minutes, 20 or 30 ml of 10% calcium gluconate (93 mg of elemental calcium/10 mL) should be given slowly. If symptoms persist, 15 mg/kg of elemental Ca should be given by continuous infusion over 4 to 6 hours.

In chronic hypoparathyroidism, one gives large daily doses of oral Ca combined with large doses of vitamin D. A dose of 2 to 4 g of oral elemental Ca (8–16 650-mg calcium carbonate tablets) is given daily. Vitamin D may be given as 50,000 to 150,000 units of vitamin D_2 a day. It is necessary to follow serum Ca and phosphate closely. One aims to achieve a nearly normal serum Ca, but without PTH, much of the Ca will be excreted in the urine.

CASE STUDY 6

Hypocalcemia in Chronic Renal Failure

A 68-year-old patient was referred to you for follow-up. He has a history of membranous glomerulonephritis, and his creatinine has been increasing for the last several months.

LABORATORY DATA

Ca 6.0 mg/dL	Phosphate 8.0 mg/dL
Creatinine 5.0 mg/dL	Albumin 2.0 Gm/dL
Urinary protein excretion 3.2g/24h	

Question 1. What effect does the hypoalbuminemia have on the serum Ca?
Question 2. How does renal failure contribute to this patient's hypocalcemia?
Question 3. How does one treat these changes caused by renal failure?
Question 4. What other factors are contributing to hypocalcemia?

1. What effect does the hypoalbuminemia have on the serum Ca?

Since 0.8 mg calcium binds to 1 g of albumin, a decrease in the serum albumin will result in a decrease in the total serum Ca, without affecting the ionized Ca. One may therefore determine a "corrected" serum Ca, which will take the hypoalbuminemia into account.

$$\text{Corrected serum Ca} = (4 - \text{serum albumin}) \times 0.8 + \text{serum Ca} \qquad \text{(Eq. 8-3)}$$

where 4 equals the normal serum albumin. Substituting in the values for our patient,

$$\text{Corrected serum Ca} = (4 - 2) \times 0.8 + 5.0 = 6.6 \qquad \text{(Eq. 8-4)}$$

This value provides only an estimation. The binding of Ca to albumin is affected by blood pH, and hypoalbuminemia may increase the Ca binding of albumin. One may therefore obtain an ionized serum Ca, which will be a more accurate assessment of Ca stores.

2. How does renal failure contribute to this patient's hypocalcemia?

Renal failure is a frequent cause of hypocalcemia. The traditional theory has been that of the "trade-off" hypothesis. Increases in serum phosphate occur because of the inability of the kidney to excrete phosphate in renal insufficiency. The increased serum phosphate causes complexation with Ca, resulting in minute decreases in ionized Ca. Hypocalcemia elicits PTH secretion, causing increased bone resorption and correction of serum Ca. The increase in PTH causes increased phosphate excretion, normalizing serum phosphate. These changes result in increased PTH levels and an increase in alkaline phosphatase, as bone resorption occurs. Calcium is gradually removed from bone, and bone pain and fractures occur.

This theory has come into question recently. It has been found that if patients were kept normocalcemic, the increase in PTH would still occur, suggesting that mild hypocalcemia is not always present when PTH increases. Recently, the important role of vitamin D has been appreciated. Decreased kidney mass and function result in reduced amounts of 1,25 alpha hydroxylase, and 1,25 OH D levels decrease markedly. The decrease in 1,25 OH D stimulates PTH secretion, even in the presence of normocalcemia. Also, 1,25 OH D causes decreased effect of PTH on the bone. Even with markedly elevated PTH levels, bone resorption may not be maximal. Therefore, elevated PTH levels resulting from decreased vitamin D cause increased bone resorption. However, in the absence of vitamin D, GI absorption of Ca is decreased, and the effect of PTH on the bone is decreased. The result is increased PTH levels, low 1,25 OH D levels, and an increased alkaline phosphatase.

3. How does one treat these changes caused by renal failure?

An important aspect of treatment is to decrease serum phosphate and restore vitamin D. The first step is dietary restriction of phosphate. Phosphate content is high in dairy products, and these agents must be avoided to a large extent. Other substances high in phosphate include chocolate, nuts, and some cola products.

Dietary restriction alone is not enough to correct hyperphosphatemia. Therefore patients are usually given oral agents that prevent GI absorption of phosphate. These medications are either Al-based or Ca-based. The Al-based agents are usually aluminum hydroxide in liquid or tablet form. These agents are given at mealtime, because it is at this time that phosphate is presented to the GI tract, and its absorption must be inhibited. Another dose is given at bedtime, as intestinal secretions of phosphate occur, and this phosphate should also be removed with aluminum hydroxide. Aluminum-based agents are the most potent binders of phosphate. However, their use is limited because chronic Al administration results in Al toxicity, which predominantly affects the central nervous system and bone. Patients may develop an irreversible dementia, and bone deposition of Al complicates renal bone disease. Aluminum may be chelated with desferoxamine, but it is highly preferable to avoid toxicity initially. Therefore, Al should only be used briefly, if at all, in the initial management of hyperphosphatemia. If hyperphosphatemia continues despite the use of other agents and a restricted diet, low doses of oral Al may be used, and the presence of Al toxicity may be monitored closely with serum Al levels, serum Al measurements after desferoxamine infusion, and bone biopsies. Of note, sucralfate contains Al and should be prescribed for only short-term use in patients with chronic renal failure.

The agents used routinely to manage hyperphosphatemia are Ca-based. The most frequently used agent is calcium carbonate, which is also given with meals and at bedtime. The over-the-counter antacid Tums is an acceptable agent, as it contains calcium carbonate. The disadvantage of calcium carbonate is that it does not bind phosphate as strongly as Al, and, when vitamin D therapy is initiated, these patients may become hypercalcemic due to increased GI calcium absorption. Newer agents may result in less Ca absorption and may become preferable alternatives for treatment of hyperphosphatemia. Calcium acetate is a medication that binds phosphate more strongly and is associated with less Ca absorption than calcium carbonate.

Once the serum phosphate is under reasonable control, one may begin treatment with 1,25 OH D. Restoration of vitamin D will decrease PTH levels and decrease bone resorption. However, vitamin D will also increase calcium and phosphate absorption from the GI tract, and one must follow serum Ca and phosphate levels extremely closely. It is preferable to keep the serum Ca in the top-normal range, and the serum phosphate in the normal range. These dietary and medication changes will frequently normalize the serum PTH, Ca, and phosphate. However, there are still patients who will not show a decline in their PTH levels. It is these patients who provide a dilemma in terms of management and suggest there are other unidentified factors at play.

4. What other factors are contributing to hypocalcemia?

Nephrotic syndrome in itself may cause hypocalcemia because of the loss of vitamin D binding proteins (with vitamin D attached) in the urine.

Also, hyperphosphatemia causes hypocalcemia directly in several ways. First, increased serum phosphate in itself decreases production of 1,25 OH D. Also, bone resorption is decreased. When the product of serum Ca and Ph (both in mg/dL) exceeds 60, precipitation of Ca and phosphate occurs in the skin, blood vessels, joints, and myocardium.

FURTHER READINGS

Agus ZS, Wasserstein A, Goldfarb S: Disorders of calcium and magnesium homeostasis. Am J Med 72: 473, 1982

Bauer W, Federman D: Hyperparathyroidism epitomized: the case of Captain Charles E. Martell. Metabolism 11(1):21, 1962

Endres DB, Villanueva R: Measurement of parathyroid hormone. Endocrin Metab Clin North Am 18(3): 611, 1989

Fitton A, McTavish D: Pamidronate: a review of its pharmacological properties and therapeutic efficacy in resorptive bone disease. Drugs 41(2):289, 1991

Gucalp R, Ritch P, Wiernik PH et al: Comparative study of pamidronate disodium and etidronate disodium in the treatment of cancer-related hypercalcemia. J Clin Onc 10(1):134, 1992

Hoffman E: The Chvostek Sign: a clinical study. Am J Surg 96:33, 1958

Hosking DJ: Assessment of renal and skeletal components of hypercalcemia. Calcified Tiss Int 46S:S11, 1990

Kelepouris E: Renal handling of calcium. Am J Nephrol 8:226, 1988

Mundy GR: Calcium Homeostasis: Hypercalcemia and Hypocalcemia. Martin Dunitz, London, 1989

Mundy GR: Incidence and pathophysiology of hypercalcemia. Calcified Tiss Int 46S:S3, 1990

Muggia FM: Overview of cancer-related hypercalcemia: epidemiology and etiology. Sem Onc 17(2)suppl. 5:3, 1990

Ralston S, Gallacher J: Cancer-associated hypercalcemia: morbidity and mortality. Ann Int Med 112:499, 1990

Warrell R, Murphy WK, Schulman P et al: A randomized double-blind study of gallium nitrate compared with etidronate for acute control of cancer-related hypercalcemia. J Clin Onc 9(8):1467, 1991

Zaloga GP: Hypocalcemic crisis. Crit Care Clin 7:191, 1991

Ziyadeh FN, Agus ZS: Effects of endocrine disease on the kidney. p. 1529. In Becker KL (ed.): Principles and Practice of Endocrinology and Metabolism. JP Lippincott, Philadelphia, 1990

Ziyadeh FN, Goldfarb S: Disorders of phosphate homeostasis. p. 2339. In: Stein JH (ed): Internal Medicine, 3rd Ed., 1990

Index

Note: Page numbers followed by f indicate figures, and those followed by t indicate tables.